Prof. D. William Molloy
Dr. Brian Daly

LET ME DECIDE

The Health and Personal Care Directive that speaks for you when you can't

"This admirable booklet gives clear and explicit instructions on how to make an advanced directive about one's healthcare. Everything is explained, everything is defined and there is practical advice on how to make one's views unequivocally clear. Every doctor should read this book." Age and Aging

First Published December 1989

26th Edition, 2017

ISBN 978-0-9935408-0-6

1. Living Will.

2. Terminally ill – Medical Care.

3. Advance Care Directive.

Published in 2017 by Newgrange Press.

Newgrange Press (Ireland), Woodstown Strand, Co. Waterford,
Y6N-36-WT8, Ireland.

Visit the *Let Me Decide* website at: www.letmedecide.ie

Design and typesetting:

Kunnert + Tierney, Cork

www.kunnertandtierney.com

Printed in Ireland.

This book is dedicated to
Prof. Cillian Twomey, a gentleman and a scholar.

LET ME PASS GENTLY

D.W.M., FEBRUARY 6, 2000

Let me pass gently into the light, for peaceful rest
at long journey's end.
Let me not struggle painfully through
a drawn out, difficult dying process
like so many before me.

Let me pass gently into the light,
like autumn leaves floating to the ground,
clouds passing behind a mountain,
or loons flying into the sun's fading embers,
slipping, silently out of sight.

Let me pass gently into the light,
in my own bed at home,
surrounded by family and fine friends,
sitting around our kitchen table,
taking turns to say goodbye.

Let me pass gently into the light,
to that vast, ineffable from which I came,
to join those who have gone before and
watch the coming generations
enjoy their time in the sun.

Let me pass gently into the light,
to take back the face I once had
before I was born,
leaving all to wonder where I am,
passed on, only in memory now.

Let me pass gently into the light,
so our children laugh about our time together,
the full days and shared intimacies,
happy that we made the best
of our short lives.

Let me pass gently into the light,
so my children smile when they think of me
and our happy times together
rather than weeping with sadness or regret
for my suffering or loss of dignity.

Let me pass gently into the light,
so I can show others how to die
naturally and peacefully,
and my death or dying does not cast
a shadow over their bright lives.

Let me pass gently into the light,
after I have made the best
of this short visit, and my opportunity to
share the wonder of our lives together,
and leave with no regrets.

LET ME DECIDE REVIEWS

"This admirable booklet gives clear and explicit instructions on how to make an advance directive about one's healthcare. Everything is explained, everything is defined, there is practical advice on how to make one's views unequivocally clear. Every doctor should read this book."

Age and Aging

"This is quite the most important book you will ever read."

Sir Dirk Bogarde

"Let Me Decide is an important and influential part of the new generation of living wills, currently being drafted and we urge every member with an interest in this area to obtain a copy and read it carefully."

Last Rights

"Overall Let Me Decide provides an excellent format and instructional guide for the drafting of advanced healthcare directives."

Geriatrics

"Thank you many times for your excellent booklet – Let Me Decide."

Margaret E. Kuhn, National Convener, Gray Panthers

"Let Me Decide, takes patients beyond a living will to a point where they can decide about specific treatments and illnesses."

Times Colonist B.C.

"Let Me Decide is an easy-to-read but comprehensive booklet."

Alzheimer Journal

"Let Me Decide is an extraordinary little book very thoughtful and extremely helpful I strongly urge you to read it and use it."

Gisele Toupin, Ontario Director General, Veterans Affairs Canada

"A major step forward in the field."

Legion

"The nice thing about Let Me Decide is that it gives the reader, in very clear and easy-to-understand language, an explanation of what is involved in various medical interventions and procedures. It is useful to read no matter what advanced directive of living will a person may end up using... the best of the lot."

Eike-Henner Kluge

"A pioneering document which is leading the way in providing patients/ clients with a guideline for facilitating decision making and recording personal preferences for healthcare. Let Me Decide is an excellent resource for healthcare professionals working with adult clients, who wish to deal with the difficult questions surrounding options for medical care in reversible and irreversible conditions."

National, Special Ethics Edition

"Let Me Decide is a masterpiece."

Dr. H. Schneiderman, Physician in Chief,
Hebrew Home and Hospital, University of Connecticut

CONTENTS

THE IMPORTANCE OF AN ADVANCE CARE DIRECTIVE – IT'S ALL ABOUT YOU

The freedom to decide **one's own destiny, is the right of every competent person.**

If we become critically ill, **we may not be able to make these decisions.**

The Let Me Decide Advance Care Directive will speak for YOU. **If you become incapacitated by disease or injury and cannot communicate for yourself.**

Let Me Decide lets **YOU take control over your life and how illness might impact YOU.**

YOU will receive the care YOU choose at the end of your life.

Your family do not have to guess what YOU would want.

YOU prevent conflict, stress, and potential lifelong regret among your loved ones.

Healthcare professionals will make decisions on your healthcare following YOUR clear and stated wishes.

FOREWORD

Prof. D. William Molloy
MB, BCh, BAO, MRCPI, FRCPC

William was born in Waterford and qualified in medicine in 1977 at University College Cork. He obtained his membership in medicine in 1981. He emigrated to Canada where he trained in Geriatrics at the Universities of Manitoba, Western Ontario, and McMaster. He was Professor of Medicine and Chair in Aging at McMaster University.

He authored and co-authored, Common Sense Geriatrics; Vital Choices; What Are We Going To Do Now? Capacity to Decide; Alzheimer's Disease; Set Me Free; The Fine Detail; SMMSE: A User's Guide; Dysfunctional Behaviour in Dementia; I Wanna Go Home, It's my life, I decide, and Let Me Pass Gently.

He returned to Ireland in 2010 to his alma mater, University College Cork, as Professor of Medicine and Chair in Gerontology and Rehabilitation. This is the twenty seventh edition of Let Me Decide.

Dr. Brian Daly
B.C.L., L.L.B., Attorney-at-Law (New York),
Solicitor (Ireland), M.B, B.Ch, B.A.O (Hons)

Brian is from Dungarvan, Co Waterford. He worked as a lawyer in San Francisco and Ireland. He returned to University College Cork to study Medicine. He has collaborated in research with William since 2012, specifically in the areas of dementia, risk assessment in the elderly, and end of life care.

1 | INTRODUCTION

I am ageing. You are ageing. The whole world is ageing because we are living longer. At the same time society is changing rapidly. The single nuclear family with mother, father and children is becoming less common. Many of us live alone or in couples without children. Even those with children are more likely to live apart from their children. More and more of us face old age without family support. This means we should plan ahead for a period of disability at the end of life. Let Me Decide was designed to let you take control of that period at the end of your life when you may not be able to decide for yourself. It extends your autonomy to a period of your life when you are most vulnerable.

The freedom to decide one's own destiny is the right of every competent person. This includes the right to accept or refuse medical treatments. Many people want to choose their own healthcare* because they have definite opinions on how they want to be treated. But if we become critically ill, we may not be able to make these decisions. We may be too sick to make our wishes known.

The purpose of this booklet is to help you take control of and record your wishes for your health and personal care for a future time, if you are unable to speak for yourself. In the future if you become incapacitated by disease or injury and cannot communicate for yourself, the *Let Me Decide* Advance Care Directive will speak for you.

Over the last fifty years, medicine has advanced at an amazing pace. What would have been considered miraculous then, is now routine. People are kept alive with heart, kidney and liver transplants. Limbs are sewn back on, and diseases that were once fatal, are cured. At the same time, modern medicine has become

all terms underlined in the text are defined in the glossary more technical, more sophisticated and more complicated. This explosion in technology in healthcare has brought about new investigations and treatments. This has added to the complexity of decisions that people face.

The general public can be overwhelmed by the amount of technology used in modern healthcare. People are confused by the jargon that health professionals use. A person can go into hospital and have an ECG, EEG, EMG, colonoscopy, laparoscopy, bronchoscopy or thousands of different tests for diseases such as SLE, COPD, or IHD. For the person with pain, shortness of breath, weight loss or tiredness, this jargon is meaningless. Blood tests and x-rays mean more needles and scans that create endless printouts and images on screens that must be interpreted by even more doctors and technicians. Decisions about tests and treatments can be overwhelming. Simple comprehensive educational tools are needed to guide patients and families through important and what might even be unexpected life and death decisions.

At the same time, through the internet, newspapers, magazines, television and film, the general public has become better educated about illnesses and treatments. Advocacy groups like the Heart and Stroke Foundation, Alzheimer Society, Cancer Society and Kidney Foundation provide more information and support. Patients and their families want to keep control over their healthcare. Many feel overwhelmed in large, modern hospitals that have morphed and evolved into vast medical-industrial complexes that can bewilder and intimidate.

Death was once something that took place at home, surrounded by family. The majority of people now die in hospital. With 'advances' in medicine, our attitude to death has changed. Death for humans is our ultimate failure. There is a belief that death can be resisted, postponed or even prevented.

Public Perception of CPR treatment success

CPR in All Settings
Perception: The general public believes that CPR is successful in approx. 60% of cases or more

Reality of CPR treatment success

CPR in Hospital Setting
Reality: Less than 20% of people survive

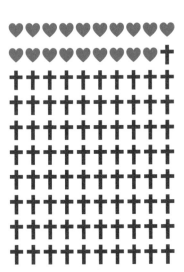

CPR in Community Setting
Reality: About 6% of people survive

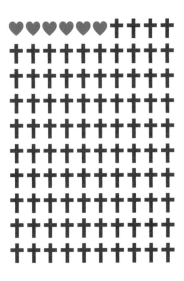

CPR in disabled older adults at end of life
Reality: No survival

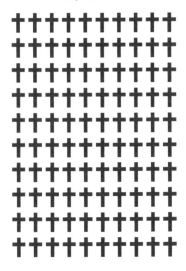

Much of the public knowledge of procedures such as Cardio-Pulmonary Resuscitation (CPR) is informed by television. CPR is a procedure that is performed on people whose heart and breathing have stopped (cardiac arrest). Recent studies have shown that the general public believes that CPR is successful in approximately 60% of cases, or more. This is similar to the success rates seen in medical dramas on TV. However, reality is very different. Less than 20% of people who have a cardiac arrest survive with CPR. Only 10% of older adults who have a cardiac arrest in hospital are still alive after one year. For those who arrest in the community, the survival is about 6% For older adults with chronic diseases survival may be closer to 0%.

CPR is not without complications, it can cause rib fractures from repeated forceful pressure on the chest, and burns to the chest from repeated shocks. Even when CPR is successful, individuals can be left with residual brain injury. The survival after CPR has changed little in the last 40 years, despite huge changes in medical practice. The likely survival is much lower for individuals with advanced disease. For people with chronic diseases at the end of life, procedures such as CPR are futile. Death will occur regardless of any treatment given or procedure performed. To quote Dame Cicely Saunders on CPR, "*If the expected outcome is death, a procedure less dignified and peaceful (as CPR) could hardly be devised.*"

People are concerned that in the event of a serious illness they may not receive the treatment they would want. They worry they may become too sick to let doctors know their wishes, or that they may not even be asked. Some fear that they will be connected to machines and kept alive in a poor, unacceptable, quality of life where treatments don't prolong life, but just drag out the dying process and prolong suffering. They fear they will be kept 'alive' in a disabled condition they would consider intolerable because of chronic confusion, suffering, loss of dignity, lacking control or independence. Some fear dying even more than death. They are concerned that their dying will be dragged out while they are in an intolerable condition that could be considered a 'state worse than death'.

Medical staff also faces a dilemma when they have to make decisions for people at the end of life. Doctors sometimes don't want to take responsibility for decisions that will affect the rest of a patient's life. Many doctors do not feel comfortable making life or death decisions for strangers they are meeting for the first time when these decisions are needed.

If you become ill or confused, family, friends or doctors must make decisions for you. These difficult decisions can present a 'no-win' situation for everyone. If members of a family ask the doctors to do 'everything' to keep a loved one alive and that person dies after weeks, months, or even years of suffering, the family may feel guilty that they put the patient through needless tests and treatments. They may feel that treatment only prolonged the patient's suffering and postponed death. On the other hand, if they let their family member 'die with dignity', they may feel later that they should have done more. Unfortunately there is no going back. These decisions, together with the uncertainty, can leave a legacy of regret, even bitterness in survivors if they feel they got it wrong.

More problems develop if family members don't agree. Some want 'everything' done to keep the person alive at all costs. Others want palliative care for symptom relief, comfort and relief of pain. Children from divorced marriages resent step-parents or common-law spouses making decisions for their parents. *The Daughter From California Syndrome* describes a situation where an adult child, who has been out of contact for years, turns up when a parent is dying, and tries to take control. This adult child demands that doctors do 'everything' to try to keep the parent alive. She feels guilty and wants to make peace with the parent. Friends and other family members, who remained in close contact, accept the parent's death. They request a palliative approach to care. The daughter who has not been in touch has not come to terms with the parent's death and plays havoc with the family and healthcare team.

Conflicts among next-of-kin over end of life treatment decisions can leave lasting resentment and even divide families forever.

We can't make clear decisions if we are sidelined by emotion, arguments and uncertainty. Doctors caught in the crossfire between feuding family members who want polar opposite treatments, are in a 'no-win' situation. They are damned if they do, and damned if they don't.

How can we protect ourselves to make sure we get the healthcare we want? How can we let others know our wishes and protect our families and friends from this dilemma?

Discussing these issues in advance can prevent conflict later. The drawback of informal discussions is that family and friends may not recall them accurately. Years later, in a time of crisis when very specific decisions must be made, the family may disagree about what the person said and meant.

If we state our wishes clearly, doctors and family don't have to second-guess what we said or what treatments we want, or do not want. Clear instructions will prevent conflict and reduce the need for 'second-guessing'. If people leave clear instructions for their health and personal care, and become too sick to decide for themselves, doctors, family and friends will know their wishes.

They will receive the treatment they want. The family is 'off the hook'. There is no conflict, no regrets, no bitterness or recriminations. The matter is settled. Everyone can focus on providing the care the person wants and not waste time and energy arguing.

➤ This small booklet lets you take control over your dying.

➤ You will get the care you want at the end of your life.

➤ You take your family off the hook.

➤ You prevent conflict, stress, and potential life-long regret among your loved ones.

➤ You take Healthcare Professionals off the hook.

It's your life – you decide.

2 | WHAT IS AN ADVANCE CARE DIRECTIVE?

It is NOT a:
- **Will** – How to dispose of property after death.
- **Power of Attorney** – Person who can manage your financial affairs on your behalf.
- **Enduring Power of Attorney** – Person who can manage your financial affairs if you become incapable. But cannot consent on your behalf to withdraw treatment e.g. CPR, Tube Feeding, Palliative Care.

An Advance Care Directive is:

A document that states your healthcare choice in the future if you become too sick to communicate them. There are 2 types of Advance Care Directives; Instructional and Proxy.

1. Instructional Advance Care Directives

This is also known as a Living Will. This document states your wishes for certain treatment e.g. CPR, tube feeding etc. in the future if you are unable to communicate your wishes.

2. Proxy Advance Care Directive

This nominates another person (called a designated decision maker, power of attorney for healthcare) who can make healthcare decisions on your behalf.

An advance directive is a written statement that expresses your wishes in advance.

The most widely used advance directive is a Will. It contains instructions to inform others how you want your possessions distributed after death.

An advance care directive deals specifically with health and personal care. It does not deal with finances or property. It is sometimes called a *Living Will*. It contains instructions about your health and personal care in case you are not able to make healthcare decisions at a later date. The *Let Me Decide* Advance Care Directive enables you to state your wishes for medical treatment and personal care, if the time comes when you are too sick to make your wishes known.

As long as you remain competent, able to consider and communicate healthcare choices, you will make these decisions for yourself. **An advance care directive is only used if you are incompetent and unable to make your wishes known.**

There are two types of advance care directives – instructional and proxy directives.

Instructional Directive (Living Will)

An *instructional directive*, states what treatments are wanted or not wanted under any given circumstances. These statements can be general or specific. The more specific the instructions, the easier it will be for family and doctors to follow. Instructional directives are also called *Living Wills*. An instructional directive is not limited to the treatment of terminal or irreversible conditions; it can also apply to curable, reversible conditions.

Proxy Directive

The person who is completing the advance care directive is called the *donor*. A proxy is a substitute or power of attorney who you (the donor) nominate to make decisions for you, if you become incapable. A *proxy directive* is the document the donor completes to name another to make decisions for his health or personal care, if he/she becomes incapable. This *proxy* has the ability to make health and personal care decisions in much the same way as a financial power of attorney can manage finances.

The *Let Me Decide* Advance Care Directive has an *instructional* and *proxy directive*. This provides double reinforcement that your wishes are followed. If your proxy is not available during a crisis, the written instructions, in the instructional part, informs healthcare providers of your wishes. The instructional part, clearly lays out what you would want for a whole variety of eventualities. If the proxy is available, then he/she can tell the healthcare team about your wishes.

History of Advance Care Directive

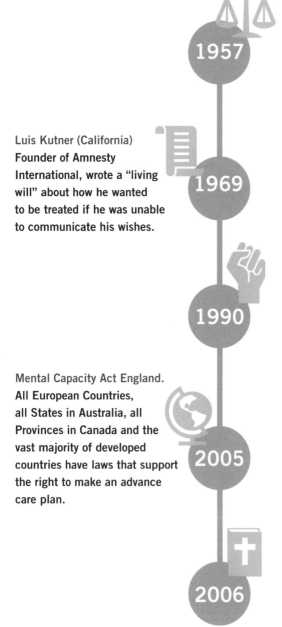

1957
Federal Hospital Law Act in Austria **allowed a person to register a care plan and the to refuse treatment if the person wishes.**

Luis Kutner (California) **Founder of Amnesty International, wrote a "living will" about how he wanted to be treated if he was unable to communicate his wishes.**
1969

1990
Patient Self Determination Act **Legalised Advance Care Directives in the USA (Federal Act-USA)**

Mental Capacity Act England. **All European Countries, all States in Australia, all Provinces in Canada and the vast majority of developed countries have laws that support the right to make an advance care plan.**
2005

2006
UN Convention on the Rights of the Person with Disabilities. **All major religions, support the right to make an Advance Care Directive. Worldwide now religions laws and international conventions support Advance Care Directives.**

3 | ARE ADVANCE CARE DIRECTIVES LEGAL?

The short answer is a resounding <u>YES</u>.

Competent adults have the right to decide what shall be done to their bodies. Any healthcare professional who treats you in a manner inconsistent with your wishes can be charged with assault and/or negligence.

The majority of European countries have legislation supporting advance care directives. In 2016, all 50 US states, Canada, Australia, New Zealand and the majority of European countries have legalized instructional directives, proxy advance directives, and Powers of Attorney. Even in the absence of legislation, advance care directives always were, and always will be supported by the common law as legally binding written documents. They safeguard a person's fundamental rights of self-determination, autonomy, bodily integrity, and privacy.

As long as the Advance Care Directive:
- Is completed voluntarily by someone with the capacity to do so
- Contains no illegal directions (for example, a direction for euthanasia)
- Has directions that are sufficiently clear to be understood by medical professionals.

An advance directive is a legally binding document that must be followed. Courts in Europe, Northern America, Australia and beyond support advance directives based on these principles.

Patients, doctors and healthcare professionals have often been under the misconception that just because advance care directives were not legislated in a certain jurisdiction, that they did not have legal standing. As a result, people were less likely to create advance care directives, and doctors less likely to follow them, for fear of legal repercussions.

As more countries pass legislation supporting advance care directives, more and more people will complete them.

Advance Care Directives – the early days

The right of competent people to control their health and personal care is long recognised. In 1914, the case of *Schloendorff v. Society of New York Hospitals*, established that a surgeon, who performs an operation, without his patient's consent, commits an assault.

Mary Schloendorff consented to an abdominal examination, under anaesthetic, to investigate a tumour, on condition that if a tumour was found, there would be no further surgery. The surgeon found a malignant tumour and removed it, contrary to her wishes. She sued the surgeon. Justice Benjamin Cardozo remarked that *"every human being, of adult years and sound mind, has a right to determine what shall be done to his own body."*

The 'Schloendorff' case established that an adult could refuse medical treatment, even if this resulted in death. This works well if a person is able to understand and communicate her wishes. Where a patient lacks the ability to understand and make decisions or has lost the ability to speak and communicate her wishes (for example, as a result of a stroke or dementia) then she is not in a position to make her wishes known.

Medical advances (such as artificial ventilators and cardio-respiratory resuscitation) mean that many 'fatal' diseases can

24

now be cured. Life can be sustained, where death would have been a certainty in the past. However, prolongation of life is not always in a person's best interests or what the person would want. While these advances were being made, there was a shift away from a paternalistic model of medicine, where doctors direct their patient's care, with little input from the patients themselves. The system moved to a more autonomous model that showed greater respect for patient autonomy. Autonomy values and encourages patient input to take an active part in decisions regarding their medical care, especially when it comes to refusing or withdrawing from medical treatments.

More and more people became concerned that the health-care system was using technology and resources inappropriately. These resources were used not to prolong life, but to drag out the dying process that meant further suffering for patients and their families. In Austria, in 1957, the *Federal Hospital Law Act* provided for the registration of an individual's medical record and the right to refuse treatment, in the event of incapacity later.

In 1969, Luis Kutner a US human rights activist, lawyer, and co-founder of Amnesty International, first proposed the concept of a living will. This was in response to the case of a young student who ended the life of his cancer-stricken mother after she asked him to end her suffering. Advance care directives (living wills) began to appear in California. People wrote out their wishes fearing that the healthcare system would treat them too aggressively and prolong their dying, when they did not have an acceptable quality of life.

Advance directives have come a long way since then. The medical profession, laws, and courts have been trying to catch up ever since. Throughout the Western world, the courts at every level have heard landmark cases involving disputes between terminally ill patients, their governments, healthcare providers, and families regarding the withholding of treatment. Almost universally, the courts rule in favour of patient autonomy over healthcare, even if that decision shortens life, and hastens death.

Legislative progression through Western world

Advance care directives have been recognised by the majority of Western jurisdictions. Countries lacking legislation are now the exception. The United States passed the *Patient Self Determination Act* in 1990, in support of advance care directives. In England, the *Mental Capacity Act* (2005), legislated for advance decisions to refuse treatment and for lasting powers of attorney, covering healthcare decisions. Finland (*Act on the Status and Rights of Patients 1992*), Denmark (*Law on Patients' Legal Status 1998*), and the Netherlands (*Medical Treatment Contracts Act 1994*) have similar statutes. There is also legislation in Portugal, Germany, Belgium, Estonia, Georgia, Hungary, Spain, Luxembourg, Ireland and Switzerland.

International Support

The international community has shown overwhelming support for advance care directives. *The European Convention on Human Rights and Biomedicine*, 1997, expressly referenced advance directives in Article 9, stating that "*the previously expressed wishes relating to a medical intervention by a patient who is not, at the time of the intervention, in a state to express his or her wishes, shall be taken into account.*" Further, Article 3 of the 2006 *UN Convention on the Rights of Persons with Disabilities (CRPD)* supports "*respect for inherent dignity, individual autonomy including the freedom to make one's own choices*" and for "*respect for difference and acceptance of persons with disabilities as part of human diversity and humanity*" to be shown.

26

Advantages of Let Me Decide from a legal perspective

As long as a directive, completed by a competent adult, is sufficiently clear, and contains no illegal directions, it is legally binding. The *Let Me Decide* directive has many features that set it apart from other advance care directives.

The language in *Let Me Decide* is very clear. It uses medical terms that leave no doubt as to what the person wants. Other directives often use vague terminology. The person completing the *Let Me Decide* directive has to learn what these terms mean. The healthcare professionals who have to follow these directives often have to make life or death decisions based on these instructions. In many cases, healthcare professionals are meeting a person for the first time when she is critically ill or dying. It is important that instructions are clear. The terms used in *Let Me Decide* are valid medical terms that are clearly defined. The directive is easily understood by those who must follow it.

It contains a space for two witnesses and the family doctor's signature. While not a requirement of some legal statutes, it is recommended that these are signed. These signatures further strengthen its legal status and the likelihood that the doctor will know about it and that it will be followed. This will ensure that the doctor or nurse explain all the terms so that there is no doubt that the patient understands the terms and their implications.

Finally, there is a section that allows for the directive to be updated, should a patient's views on their healthcare, or circumstances, change.

These features ensure that *Let Me Decide*, if completed correctly, will be enforceable in any jurisdiction, whether advance care directives are legislated for or not.

Let Me Decide has been used in many countries and has been studied more than any other advance directive.

4 | THE LET ME DECIDE ADVANCE CARE DIRECTIVE OVERVIEW

7 Steps to complete Let Me Decide Advance Care Directive

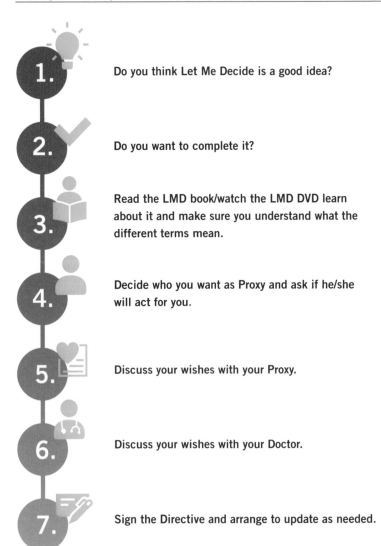

1. Do you think Let Me Decide is a good idea?

2. Do you want to complete it?

3. Read the LMD book/watch the LMD DVD learn about it and make sure you understand what the different terms mean.

4. Decide who you want as Proxy and ask if he/she will act for you.

5. Discuss your wishes with your Proxy.

6. Discuss your wishes with your Doctor.

7. Sign the Directive and arrange to update as needed.

The *Let Me Decide* Advance Care Directive uses medical terms that have definite and clear meaning so that doctors and families can interpret your instructions clearly. If you want to use the *Let Me Decide* directive, you must first learn what these terms mean. The Directive provides a wide range of treatment options. You can choose different treatments, depending on whether you would consider your condition acceptable, or irreversible and intolerable. You can choose treatment for a life threatening illness, if you can't eat, or if your heart stops (cardiac arrest). You can also state what level of disability you would find acceptable or unacceptable. A glossary is provided at the back that explains each of the terms.

The *Let Me Decide* Advance Care Directive has five sections. Each section is explained below.

1. Introduction

This section states the reasons why you want to complete this directive. It advises others that the directive should not be used if you are able to make decisions for yourself. It should only be used if you are incapacitated by disease or injury and unable to make your own decisions. It revokes previous documents and establishes this document as the latest expression of your wishes.

2. Personal Statement

This section contains your personal statement where you state what level of disability you would find unacceptable.

An introductory phrase: "*I would consider an unacceptable condition to be any condition…*" is completed in your own words to tell others what level of disability you would consider unacceptable. Try to state your wishes as clearly as possible.

You are provided with a menu of possible disabilities (e.g. in a permanent coma, unable to recognize family or friend's, unable to walk, bed bound etc.). You can say whether you would find each disability acceptable or unacceptable when you personalize your directive.

The personal statement can be used to cover a whole range of issues. You can state your wishes for personal care, such as where you live, safety issues, clothing and hygiene. You can also make your wishes known about blood transfusions, cremation and organ donation.

It is very important to discuss your wishes with your proxy so that he/she knows what you want.

3. Healthcare Chart

This chart documents your wishes for treatment of life-threatening illness, cardiac arrest and feeding, depending on whether your condition is acceptable or unacceptable.

We recommend that you review your Directive with your doctor every year or so. Space is provided for these updates. If, on review, you make no changes, just write *"No Change"*, sign and date it with your doctor. If you change your wishes, you should tell your proxy and family doctor. Update all the copies of the directive and have everybody sign them. It is a good idea to review your choices and sign your statement after an admission to hospital, after a significant illness or change in your health, so that your directive is current and your choices aren't questioned later.

4. Definitions

This section contains explanations of terms used in the Directive. The glossary at the back provides explanations and descriptions of other medical terms.

5. Naming Others (Family Doctor, Power of Attorney/Proxy and Witnesses)

This section contains the names, addresses and telephone numbers of your family doctor, proxy(s) and witnesses. Home and work numbers are given, along with additional numbers where they can be reached in an emergency.

Witnesses who sign this section can be anyone except the following:

- A close family member of the person completing the Directive
- Anyone who might expect to receive a financial benefit from the estate of the person
- The proxy
- The proxy's spouse or child (natural or adopted)
- Anyone who is less than 18 years old.

Witnesses should have no reason to believe that the person filling out the directive is incapable of understanding of giving instructions, or is being put under pressure to make choices, other than their own.

Now let's consider what we mean by acceptable and irreversible/unacceptable disability.

Level of Independence/Dependence

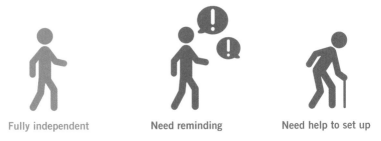

Fully independent   Need reminding   Need help to set up

Examples of Self-Directed Activities

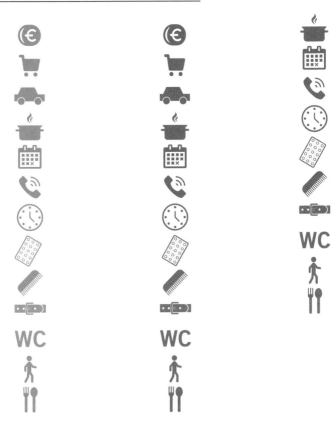

Figure 5.1: Different levels of disability and their consequences on independence.

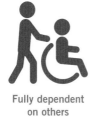

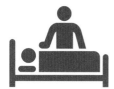

Needs assistance

**Fully dependent
on others**

**Need 24 hour
supervision and care**

WC

Progression over time from health and independence to disability with an unacceptable quality of life:

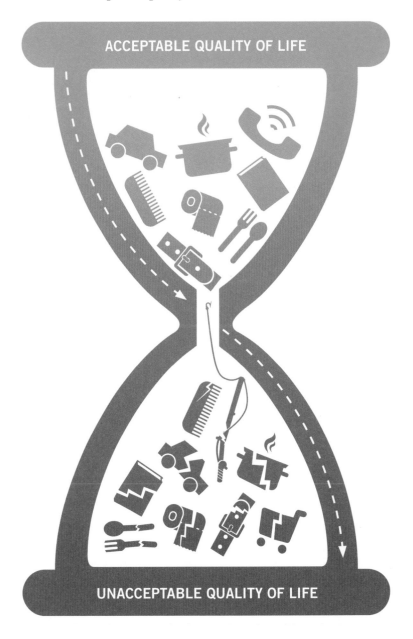

5 | IRREVERSIBLE/UNACCEPTABLE AND ACCEPTABLE CONDITIONS

Advancing age or chronic illnesses can bring progressive disability with loss of independence and quality of life. **Figure 5.1** shows a range of functions we all perform daily and the consequences to our independence and quality of life if we lose the ability to perform these activities. At a certain point a disability may become unacceptable. This is the threshold where a person thinks, "*I would accept this, but I would not accept that.*" The purpose of the Personal Statement is to allow you to describe what you consider unacceptable and make treatment choices accordingly. It is important to consider carefully what you would consider acceptable and unacceptable.

    Figure 5.2 shows roughly how your treatment choices will vary depending on your level of disability, independence and quality of life. For example, if you are fully independent, you might request that 'everything' be done to preserve life, if you had a life threatening illness, (like a bleeding ulcer or severe pneumonia), that was completely curable.

    However, if you were chronically ill, disabled, confused, fully dependent for washing, dressing and grooming and unable to control bladder and bowels, you might just want comfort measures or palliative care, if you developed a life threatening illness.

    Figures 5.1 and 5.2 show the progression over time from health and independence to disability with an unacceptable quality of life. It also provides likely treatment choices depending on whether your quality of life is acceptable or unacceptable.

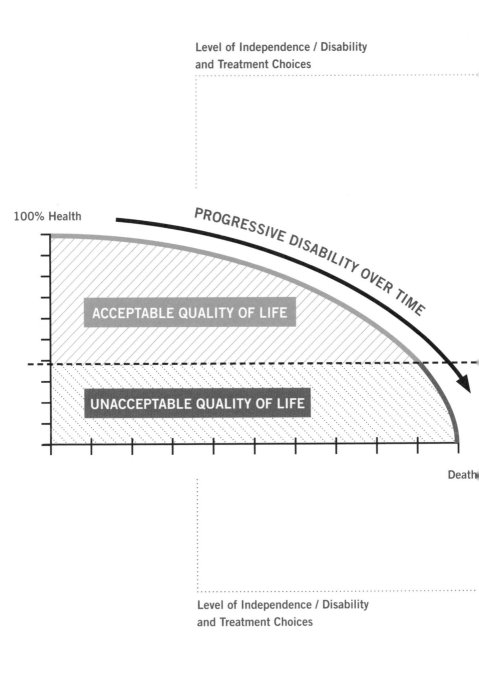

Level of Independence / Disability
and Treatment Choices

100% Health

PROGRESSIVE DISABILITY OVER TIME

ACCEPTABLE QUALITY OF LIFE

UNACCEPTABLE QUALITY OF LIFE

Death

Level of Independence / Disability
and Treatment Choices

Figure 5.2: Threshold between Acceptable and Unacceptable
Disability and associated treatment choices.

ACCEPTABLE QUALITY OF LIFE

Examples for an acceptable quality of life:
- Active
- Independent
- Self-determining
- Engaged

Active Treatment to preserve life

Use Feeding Tube   Do CPR   Intensive Care

UNACCEPTABLE QUALITY OF LIFE

Examples for an unacceptable quality of life:
- Condition is irreversible
- Dependent for care
- Needs help with basic care
- Unable to communicate / Unable to recognise family
- Constantly confused, unable to communicate basic needs
- Incontinent, stool and urine
- Persistent vegetative state

Treatment aimed not at preserving life, but at symptom control

No Feeding Tube   No CPR   Comfort Care

Irreversible and Unacceptable Conditions

When a disability is permanent, there is no possibility of a complete recovery. Chronic diseases such as Alzheimer's, Parkinson's and certain incurable cancers are examples of irreversible illnesses that eventually lead to permanent disability, and death. People accept and deal with disability in very different ways. Some people would not consider themselves disabled if they were confined to a wheelchair or even bedridden. Others would consider this an unacceptable loss of independence. Consider how these illnesses would impair your independence and ability to carry out everyday activities such as walking, dressing, talking and eating. Consider how a disability would affect your quality of life. Describe the level of disability you would find unacceptable when you define an irreversible/unacceptable state, in your personal statement.

Acceptable Disability

If Beethoven had gone blind instead of deaf, he still could have heard his music. Blindness would have had less impact on him than deafness. But a painter like Picasso would dread blindness much more than deafness. The same disabilities can affect people in very different ways.

If you have an acceptable disability, you have an acceptable quality of life. If you had a good quality of life and developed a life-threatening illness such as a bleeding ulcer or pneumonia that could be cured with treatment, leaving no lasting disability, how would you want to be treated? In this case you might want investigations and treatments that you would not want in an intolerable/unacceptable state.

For example, you might want antibiotics for pneumonia if you were fit and healthy. You might reject antibiotics if you were in an intolerable/unacceptable state that was irreversible. Since each person would accept different irreversible disabilities, it's important to state in advance, what you would or would not accept. Consider what loss of function you would consider acceptable or unacceptable. Don't think in terms of specific illnesses. Think in terms of independence, function and quality of life. When you decide what you consider acceptable and intolerable or unacceptable, choose the level of care you would want in each case.

6 | LIFE-THREATENING ILLNESS

A life-threatening illness can potentially cause death. A healthy person who develops pneumonia would want to be vigorously treated. People with chronic diseases may be so weak that they have no resistance to fight pneumonia. People with chronic illnesses such as Parkinson's, Alzheimer's or cancer, often die from pneumonia when they are too weak to swallow or cough, if the food goes down into their lungs. A person who is already dying from an incurable illness may wish to allow pneumonia to run its course. In this condition, a person might not want antibiotics. Comfort Care may be more appropriate to relieve suffering and maintain comfort.

If a decision is made to treat an acute life-threatening illness in a dying patient, more tests and investigations may be required. This means more needles, x-rays, and intravenous lines. These procedures can be uncomfortable and painful. Treatment may not be successful and only serve to prolong the dying process. Doctors may advise families, in these cases, to allow the person to die peacefully, to prevent the patient from suffering more. Comfort or palliative care aims to relieve symptoms, keep the person comfortable and relieve pain. The goal is not to cure or extend life, but comfort and relief from suffering.

For this reason, pneumonia has been called 'an old man's friend'. It allows a dying person to go peacefully, without further suffering. For a life threatening illness, you can choose from four levels of care: comfort/supportive, limited, surgical, and intensive.

Comfort or Supportive Care

 At this level of care, tests are done and treatments given, not to prolong life, but to maintain comfort. The aim of treatment is to relieve pain and keep the person comfortable and pain-free.

Patients who have requested comfort/supportive care might have surgery, if that was necessary to improve their comfort or relieve pain. For example, if you broke a hip and had requested comfort/supportive care, surgery could be performed to pin the hip, if this was the most effective way to relieve the pain.

Similarly, antibiotics might be prescribed, if they were necessary to improve comfort. If you had a bladder or skin infection that was causing discomfort, you would receive antibiotics. You would receive oxygen if it made your breathing easier.

If you had bleeding in the stomach or intestine, you would not receive blood transfusions or drugs to stop the bleeding. If you were at home, you would be transferred to hospital for tests or treatments, only if you could not be kept comfortable in your home.

Medications and treatments are reviewed and may be stopped or modified. Certain drugs like blood thinners, aspirin to prevent stroke or cholesterol lowering pills might be stopped. Aspirin and cholesterol lowering pills are given to prevent illnesses later. They are not given for symptoms like shortness of breath or pain. The person will not notice any change if they are stopped. The healthcare team will discuss this with you if you are capable. If you are not capable, the doctors will discuss with your proxy or follow your wishes laid out in the directive.

Limited Care

 This level includes more treatment than 'comfort/ supportive', but less than 'surgical'. For example, if you developed pneumonia, you could receive antibiotics, blood tests, intravenous fluids, x-rays and oxygen. If you had bleeding from the stomach or intestine, you could receive blood transfusions and drugs to stop the bleeding.

You would not receive emergency surgery to stop the bleeding or medical tests that required a general anaesthetic. You would not be put on life-support machines. You would not go on a kidney machine (for dialysis) if your kidneys failed. If you were at home when you became ill, you could be transferred to hospital if enough care could not be provided at home.

Surgical Care

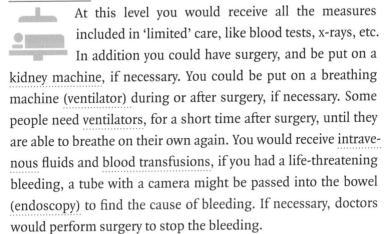 At this level you would receive all the measures included in 'limited' care, like blood tests, x-rays, etc. In addition you could have surgery, and be put on a kidney machine, if necessary. You could be put on a breathing machine (ventilator) during or after surgery, if necessary. Some people need ventilators, for a short time after surgery, until they are able to breathe on their own again. You would receive intravenous fluids and blood transfusions, if you had a life-threatening bleeding, a tube with a camera might be passed into the bowel (endoscopy) to find the cause of bleeding. If necessary, doctors would perform surgery to stop the bleeding.

You would not be transferred to intensive care, unless that was necessary to keep you comfortable. You would be transferred from home to hospital, without hesitation, for surgical care, if it was necessary.

Intensive Care

 At this level, everything a modern hospital has to offer is used to maintain life. This includes surgery, biopsies and life-support systems (kidney machines, breathing machines), and transplant surgery, if necessary (including heart, kidney, liver or bone-marrow transplants). If you were at home, you would be transferred to hospital. If you were in a small community hospital, you could be transferred to a larger hospital for a wider range of diagnostic tests and treatments. It is important to remember that just because you request intensive care – you might not necessarily receive it – either because you do not require it, would not benefit from it, or it is not available.

You will not automatically receive your chosen level of care for every illness. For example, if you asked for intensive care for a life-threatening illness, you would not automatically be admitted to intensive care every time you became ill. If admitted to hospital with a bleeding ulcer, for example, you might not necessarily require intensive care. Intensive care will only be provided, if beds are available and your condition meets the criteria for admission set out by the unit.

Let Me Decide does not allow people to demand treatment, especially if they are not needed or available. Treatments are given depending on need and availability.

7 | FEEDING

When people with severe illnesses are not able to feed themselves, a decision must be made as to how they will be fed. If they are unconscious and can't swallow, they require fluids and food artificially to maintain life. People may be unable to swallow following a stroke, from cancer, after trauma, surgery or from a variety of other causes. There are two ways to feed people who cannot feed themselves: *Basic* and *Tubes*.

Basic

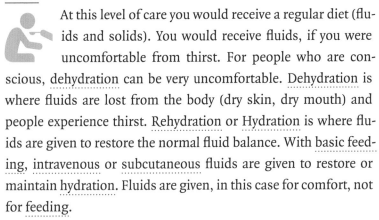 At this level of care you would receive a regular diet (fluids and solids). You would receive fluids, if you were uncomfortable from thirst. For people who are conscious, dehydration can be very uncomfortable. Dehydration is where fluids are lost from the body (dry skin, dry mouth) and people experience thirst. Rehydration or Hydration is where fluids are given to restore the normal fluid balance. With basic feeding, intravenous or subcutaneous fluids are given to restore or maintain hydration. Fluids are given, in this case for comfort, not for feeding.

Supplements and a modified diet (blended, soft, thickened food) would also be given if necessary. For instance, you may be able to swallow solids, but not liquids, or vice versa. You could be given high-energy supplements, vitamins or a modified diet. This level does not include tubes or intravenous feeding.

To maintain hydration, fluids can be given directly into the veins with *intravenous* lines. Fluids can also be given through tiny needles placed under the skin (*subcutaneous*), on the abdomen. These needles need to be changed every few days. It is not possible to feed people through subcutaneous tubes.

Tubes

(a) Intravenous Feeding

If the gut is not absorbing food, there is no point giving food by mouth or into the stomach. In this case only intravenous feeding can sustain life. *Intravenous feeding* is used for people whose gut is not absorbing food.

Intravenous means that fluids and food are given directly into the veins. The needles required for intravenous feeding eventually damage the veins. When the veins in the arms can no longer be used, larger veins nearer the heart, or in the chest and neck, are used. Intravenous lines can be inserted into the large veins near the heart, using minor procedures under local anaesthetic. Using these larger veins, called 'central lines', it is possible to give food and fluids directly into the circulation. This method of feeding is called Total Parenteral Nutrition.

(b) Stomach Tubes – Nasogastric and/or Gastrostomy Tubes

If you can't swallow and your gut is working and absorbing normally, food can be given directly into the stomach using nasogastric tubes. Nasogastric tubes are soft plastic tubes passed through the nose into the stomach. They are used for people who can digest food but can't swallow. Most people tolerate them well. Some find them uncomfortable and tend to pull them out.

Gastrostomy tubes are passed through the skin in the abdomen, directly into the stomach. When a person needs feeding for a long time, this method is preferable to a nasogastric tube.

Gastrostomy tubes can be surgically installed without a general anaesthetic, but with mild sedation. Once they are in place, they are fairly painless and trouble-free. People can bathe and shower with them. They can provide enough food and fluids to sustain people who can't swallow.

8 | CARDIO-PULMONARY RESUSCITATION (CPR)

Cardio-Pulmonary Resuscitation (CPR) is an emergency procedure that attempts to restore breathing and heartbeat in a person whose heart or breathing, or both, have stopped. Because it is an emergency when the heart or breathing stops, there is no time to contact people to discuss the situation. Decisions about CPR should be made in advance, if possible.

CPR involves external cardiac massage (pumping on the chest to push blood through the heart) and mouth-to-mouth breathing. It may also include the use of drugs, electric defibrillators (machines to shock the heart into action) or a breathing machine (mechanical ventilation).

CPR was originally developed for healthy people whose hearts had stopped from a heart attack or drowning. If a healthy person's heart stops (cardiac arrest), there is about a 20% chance of reviving that person. CPR can give this person many extra years of life. The chances of successful resuscitation vary depending on the cause of the cardiac arrest, if it is witnessed, who witnesses it and where it happens. When people have a cardiac arrest in the community, only about 6% are successfully resuscitated. People have a better chance if cardiac arrest is witnessed and resuscitation begins immediately. If people are found some time after their heart has stopped, it is unlikely they will be successfully resuscitated.

CPR nearly always fails to revive chronically ill older adults, whose heart stops after a long illness. The few who are resuscitated with CPR often do not live very long. In acute care hospitals today, medical staff usually do everything possible to save a person's life. Unless clear instructions are given to the contrary, patients are given CPR.

A No CPR order means that no attempt will be made to revive a person whose breathing or heart, or both, have stopped. Orders like these are becoming more common, particularly for people with a poor quality of life. Many fear that medical technology will be used to prolong life artificially, and keep them suspended, helplessly in a twilight zone, severely disabled in a 'state worse than death'. Many want a peaceful end to their lives and don't want to die with strangers pumping on their chests or giving them electric shocks, in a futile attempt to revive them, when they are dying, or even dead.

You need to consider whether you would want CPR if your heart stopped. If your wishes are known in advance, those who want CPR will receive it, and those who don't, will not.

You can decide, in advance, about CPR and record your wishes in the Health and Personal Care Chart.

9 | PERSONAL CARE ISSUES

If we become ill, weak or confused, others need to assist us with our personal care. We may require assistance with grooming, dressing, feeding, toilet, shopping or choosing where to live. The proxy nominated in the *Let Me Decide* directive can help with decisions about your personal care if you become incapable and if this becomes necessary. You may want to discuss these issues with your proxy, and tell your proxy about your wishes for personal care so he/she will know what you would want.

Shelter

"Promise you will never put me in a nursing home"

A parent who gets a child to make this promise, or a child who makes this promise, is creating a recipe for disaster. Sometimes it just becomes impossible to keep a parent or loved one at home. The burden of care may simply become too heavy for the family.

People who are severely confused often have no insight into their care requirements. Many believe they are still independent, even when they are unable to care for themselves. Before you ask your family to make such promises, consider this. You have become so confused that you cannot wash, dress or feed yourself. You do not recognize your family members; you have lost control of your bladder and bowels. You do not recognize your own home. You wander away and become violent when your family and caregivers try to take you home again. In this condition, would you expect your family to continue to care for you at home?

People like this can place an intolerable burden on their family members and friends. Sometimes, in spite of their best intentions, it's just not possible for family to keep a person at home.

Parents who get a spouse or children to promise to keep them at home, no matter what, set their family up for a lifetime of guilt and regret when they have no choice but to place them in a nursing home. The family feels that they have failed, betrayed their loved one, because they did not keep the promise.

Don't make unreasonable demands on your caregivers and family.

It's better to say, *"I want to stay in my home as long as possible. Do not put me in a nursing home if you can still keep me at home. I would prefer to live six months in my own home than three years in a nursing home. Keep me at home as long as possible and only transfer me to a nursing home, if I am a danger to others, or if my care becomes unmanageable at home."*

Please be careful how you use the word *"never"* in your personal statement.

Nutrition

Some people have special food preferences for religious or personal reasons. You can discuss this with your proxy and state your wishes in your personal statement. Some people are transferred to nursing homes because they are losing weight and not eating properly at home. Many old people do not eat a balanced diet and live on 'tea and toast'. Would you want to be transferred to a nursing home if you were not eating a proper diet and losing weight at home? Other decisions about feeding are covered in the Feeding section of the *Let Me Decide* Directive.

Safety

Safety issues arise at home when people have physical problems or memory loss, that put them at risk of falls, injuries or fire from smoking or cooking.

They may be at risk of wandering and getting injured or lost. They may also be at risk from skipping medications or taking too many at one time. Some steps, like disconnecting the stove, providing Meals-on-Wheels or installing a personal alarm may reduce risk. Fear for safety often leads family members to move the person to a nursing home.

Usually it comes down to a judgment call as to how much risk the person, family and caregivers can tolerate if the person stays at home. A statement such as the following may help. *"I will accept a risk of injury or even death to be able to stay in my own home. Only move me to a nursing home if I'm a danger to others."* Another person might say, *"I want to be safe and if I am not safe at home, please move me to a nursing home"* or, *"Please move me to a nursing home if the burden becomes too great on my family."*

Clothing and Hygiene

If you have preferences for clothing, for religious or personal reasons, you can use the Personal Statement to express them. You can discuss these issues with your proxy.

Many older confused people resist regular bathing and showers. If you wish, you may want to make a statement that you would only wish to be washed if your personal hygiene became offensive to others or a risk to your health.

10 | THE PERSONAL STATEMENT

Here are some disabilities that people find unacceptable.

"This is the disability I would find unacceptable. If I had this disability, I would want ..."

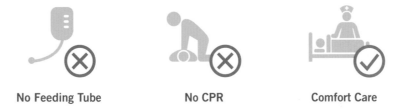

| No Feeding Tube | No CPR | Comfort Care |

Examples of Unacceptable Condition or Disabilities

Severe Dementia
- Unable to recognise family
- Incontinent of urine and stool because of lack of awareness of bowel and bladder.

Activities of daily living
- Unable to wash
- Unable to dress
- Unable to feed myself
- Unable to get from bed to chair.

Mobility
- Bed Bound
- Need people to help me get from bed to chair
- Unable to stand.

Communication
- Unable to communicate basic needs
- Unable to follow simple instructions.

Describe something real and specific, for example:
- Unable to Walk
- Unable to recognise family
- Incontinent of urine and stool
- Poor symptom control eg pain, nausea, vomiting, weakness, lethargy, shortness of breath, etc.

All of these are real and anyone can tell clearly if you have any of these conditions.

The personal statement describes a condition that is irreversible that you would find intolerable. In this irreversible and intolerable condition, you would not want treatments to prolong your life.

People have different ideas about what disabilities and medical treatments they consider unacceptable. Some would not want to be resuscitated if they were paralysed. Others fear losing bowel or bladder control. Some would not want to live in an institution, and others would not want to be tube fed. Others would not tolerate being washed and fed by others.

It is important to state as clearly as possible what conditions you would consider intolerable. Follow these simple rules when you draft your Personal Statement.

Rules for Personal Statements

- **Do not name diseases.** You could have a tiny skin cancer that is burned off and recover
- Alzheimer's. e.g. you could have a very mild case and be fully independent with just some forgetfulness
- **Consider and/or**
- If you cannot wash **and** dress **and** feed myself independently

- You have to have **all three** to be in an unacceptable condition
- If I cannot wash **or** dress **or** feed myself, this means that **any** of these three put you in an unacceptable condition.

All of these are real and anyone can tell clearly if you are in this condition.

Don't Name Diseases

When you describe this intolerable condition, do not say, "If I had *Alzheimer's disease or cancer.*" You could have skin cancer that was completely curable. Many people with early Alzheimer's experience only minor problems with memory and can still live independently. They can shop, cook and drive. Describe a level of functioning you consider intolerable in terms of everyday living. Don't name diseases, because there are great variations in the disabilities that these diseases cause.

Consider 'And' and 'Or'

When you list conditions, use the words *'and'* and *'or'* carefully. This statement: *"I would consider my condition intolerable if I can't wash and dress and feed myself"* is very different from, *"If I can't wash or dress or feed myself."* When *'and'* is used in the first statement, all three situations must be present, before your condition is intolerable. When *'or'* is used, any one of the three makes your condition intolerable.

If I have less than six months to live

Be careful using statements like, *"If I am terminally ill or have less than six months to live."* I have met lots of people who were still alive many years after they were given *"six months to live."* It's often very difficult to predict how long people with serious illnesses will live.

Describe Everyday Functions

"If the time ever comes when I am unable to dress myself, or recognize my family, or if I am so confused that I lose control over my bladder or bowel and there is no hope of recovery, then I would consider that to be an intolerable condition." This is a good statement because any illness that causes permanent disability or injury that limits your independence and freedom is covered.

It is better to say, *"If the time ever comes when I am unable to wash, dress or feed myself,"* or, *"If I can't speak to my family or make my wishes known and there is no hope of recovery,"* or, *"If my family can't care for me at home and I must live in an institution."*

Consider these conditions when you prepare your statement:

- Permanent Coma (persistent vegetative state)
- Severe Dementia i.e need help with basic care like washing dressing and feeding
- Unable to recognize the family
- Unable to communicate basic needs
- Incontinent of urine and bowels because of confusion
- Unable to dress/groom
- Need to be spoon fed
- Paralyzed on one side
- Need to be lifted in and out of bed or chair
- Unable to walk alone
- Blind
- Deaf
- Incurable cancer i.e. cancer that has spread & cannot be cured.

When you define the condition you consider intolerable, consider the level of care you would want in that condition. If you don't want certain medical procedures, for religious or other reasons, put this in your statement. If you have preferences about how you would like to be buried or cremated, you can also use the personal statement for that purpose. If a condition is irreversible/intolerable, most people request comfort/palliative care, no CPR and no tube (basic) in this state.

Some examples of personal statements are included below for your guidance.

Examples of Personal Statements

Example No 1

Joanne is 79 years old, recently widowed. She has no immediate family and lives alone in her own home. She is in good health at the moment, but this could change at any time.

Joanne is fully independent and enjoys a good quality of life now. If she got sick now and developed a life-threatening illness, she would want CPR if she had a cardiac arrest. If she develops a life-threatening illness now she would want surgical care, but no ICU. She would like basic feeding if she could not eat on her own. She would not want tube feeding.

Joanne has told her proxy that she would consider an intolerable condition: "*Dementia where I could not recognise family or communicate basic needs, if I was so confused that others had to wash and dress me or if I had a stroke or other illness that caused me to lose my speech, paralysed one side or left me permanently unable to wash, dress or feed myself.*" In this condition I would want palliative care and basic feeding only, no tubes or intravenous feeding, and I would want No CPR if I had a cardiac arrest in this condition.

Joanne wants to stay in her own home as long as possible, but she does not want to put others at risk. Joanne has indicated her healthcare choices, for an acceptable and unacceptable condition, in her Healthcare Chart and has discussed them with her proxy. Her Personal Statement continues:

"I want to stay at home as long as possible. Do not put me in a nursing home if I am not eating, washing, grooming or keeping my house clean. I can accept personal risk of wandering, falling or injuring myself. I do not want to put others at risk. If I am putting others at risk (e.g. by causing a fire) or my care becomes too much for my family and friends, then I would go into a nursing home. I would never want to be physically restrained for my own safety. If my organs can be used for others – please feel free to use them after I am dead."

Example No. 2

Paul is a 74 year old, who lives alone and has prostate cancer. The cancer has spread to his spine and local lymph glands. He is aware that as his disease progresses he will become less active and independent. He told his proxy that he cannot accept being totally bedridden and dependent on others for personal care, such as washing, dressing or feeding.

At the present time, he has an acceptable quality of life, he would want surgical care for a life-threatening illness, and CPR in the event of a cardiac arrest. He would want special diets, intravenous fluids and feeding tubes, if necessary. His Personal Statement reads as follows:

"I would consider an intolerable/unacceptable condition to be any condition, where I am unable to recognize family or communicate my basic needs, or that left me bedridden and dependent on others for personal care such as washing, dressing or feeding. If I had poor pain control, I would consider this unacceptable. I will go to a nursing home

when I can't manage at home anymore. I would not accept physical restraints for my safety, only to protect others. Let me eat what I ask for, even if it is not the best for my health. Don't ever force me to be bathed or groomed against my will. When I die, if my organs can be used for others, please go ahead and use them. I want to be cremated."

If he is in an unacceptable condition, he wants palliative care, No CPR and basic feeding.

Example No. 3

Sarah is a 35-year-old nurse who has two young children. She has a good quality of life and is in an acceptable condition. At this point, if she developed any life-threatening illness, she would want intensive care if necessary. If she had a cardiac arrest she would want CPR. She would want basic feeding, but no tube or intravenous feeding. She would accept intravenous fluids for comfort – for example, if it were given to treat dehydration.

She considers a condition unacceptable if she were no longer able to function independently. In this condition she would want comfort/palliative care. As long as she has use of her hands and can look after herself, she would accept this. She can accept paraplegia (paralysed from the waist down). She would not accept quadriplegia (paralysed all four limbs), or a stroke that significantly affected her speech, left her incontinent or needed others to wash and dress her. Her Personal Statement reads as follows:

"I would consider a condition unacceptable if I am unable to wash or dress myself, or unable to speak, or was quadriplegic. If I am so confused that I am unable to recognize family, incontinent of urine and stool, and others had to dress, groom and feed me, I would consider this unacceptable.

I would not consider paraplegia unacceptable. I would only accept a nursing home if my care became too much for my family. I would accept temporary restraints for my safety. I wish to be kept clean; I want to wear street clothes (not nightgowns) during the day. Please include me in all festivities, parties and activities if possible. After death, I agree to donate my organs to others if they can be of any use. I want to be buried, not cremated."

In this state, she would want comfort/palliative care and basic feeding and No CPR. She would want a painless death – peaceful and quiet – no blood work, no IV, no x-rays, no scans and no tube feeding.

She would not mind a post mortem, and would donate any organs if they could be used for others.

Example No. 4

Bill is a 60-year-old with chronic bronchitis. He has been in hospital three times this year already. On the last occasion he was put on a breathing machine (ventilator). Now he can't walk ouside his house because he gets so short of breath. He is happy now but does not want things to get much worse.

If he gets sick again, he wants antibiotics, inhalers and oxygen by mask. He does not want to be put on the breathing machine (ventilator) again. His main fear is that he would not be able to get off the breathing machine and would be stuck on it. If he has a cardiac arrest, he would want No CPR. If he can't eat, he would want an intravenous line and basic feeding. He does not want any feeding tubes. This is his Personal Statement:

"I would consider a condition unacceptable if I am unable to walk alone or take care of myself and had no hope of recovery. I do not want to be put on a breathing machine again. I will accept a nursing home when my wife can't cope with me at home anymore. I want to continue drinking alcohol with my meals. Please attend to my personal care, such as washing, dressing and grooming. I would not accept physical restraints

except to protect others. I agree to organ donation, and would like to be buried, not cremated."

Example No. 5

Jack is a 65-year-old retired executive. He loved golf and hill walking. Four years ago he had a heart attack and last year he had bypass surgery. Now he has angina when he climbs stairs, and sometimes wakes up short of breath. The doctors have told him that he cannot have any more surgery, and only has about 20% heart function.

Last time he was in hospital, he had a cardiac arrest and was resuscitated with CPR. He knows that he could go at anytime. Should he have another heart attack, he would not want to be resuscitated, (no CPR) and he does not want any more surgery. If he goes into heart failure again he would want limited care. He does not want to go into the intensive care unit. He does not want tube feeding, if he ever became unconscious or unable to eat. This is Jack's Personal Statement:

"I would consider a condition to be unacceptable if I am unable to walk, dress or take care of myself. I would accept a nursing home if my care becomes too difficult for my wife and family. I'm a strict vegetarian and I don't want any meat or fish. But continue to give me lots of fresh fruit, vegetables and chocolate. I would accept physical restraints for my own and others' safety. I agree to organ donation after death."

Example No. 6

Dave is a 35-year-old man with AIDS. He has been in the hospital three times this year and has lost fifty pounds since his illness began. If he becomes ill again he wants intravenous antibiotics, but he does not want intensive care. He does not want any tube feeding and he does not want a breathing machine (ventilator).

If he has a cardiac arrest, he does not want CPR. He does not want to die with people pumping his chest. Dave wrote this personal statement:

"I would consider a condition unacceptable if I am permanently confined to bed and have to spend most of my time in hospital. Thank you for all your care — I deeply appreciate it. Do everything to avoid hospitalization. I would like to die at home if at all possible. Never restrain me physically for any reason, unless I am a danger to others. Keep me comfortable at all costs; I do not want to suffer. Use whatever means are necessary to keep me comfortable. I do not want to go to the intensive care unit again. I do not want tube feeding. I would accept intravenous fluids and intravenous antibiotics. I do not want CPR if my heart stops."

11 | HOW TO COMPLETE THE LET ME DECIDE ADVANCE (LMDAD) DIRECTIVE

Introduction

The *Let Me Decide* Advance Directive (LMDAD) offers a fixed menu of choices for three outcomes – cardiac arrest, life treatment illness and inability to swallow. When first seen, the chart can seem complicated. This simple approach explains the LMDAD and explains how you can complete it with the least amount of difficulty.

Choose a Proxy or Substitute Decision-Maker

You may choose anyone you wish as your proxy. Select someone you trust who understands your wishes and respects your decisions in this matter. You can name a second person as an alternate proxy if you wish.

Authority of a Proxy

Your proxy has authority to make decisions for you about any health and personal care issues if you are mentally incapable of making decisions for yourself. You are also telling your doctors that you would like them to discuss your healthcare with your proxy if you become incapable. Your proxy can discuss healthcare decisions that you would normally make for yourself, and can tell doctors what your wishes would be, on your behalf.

Completing the Directive

When you are completing the directive, take your time, ask questions and discuss any issues that come up. Discuss the issues with the healthcare proxy(ies) and family members. Don't rush. Take your time. It may take several sessions to get through the information needed to complete the directive. You can reschedule a follow up meeting when you have had enough time to discuss with friends and family.

Never make choices because others believe they are 'appropriate' for you. Make the choices that are consistent with your values and goals.

Go over the directive, section by section, at a pace you can manage. You are in charge. Don't rush.

There are three sections where you make choices i.e. cardiac arrest, life threatening illness and tube feeding. When you understand the treatment choices for these three sections, consider what you would want now if you became so ill you could not make your wishes known.

When you understand each section, you can complete the directive.

Figure 1 shows that as we age many of us develop conditions that reduce our vitality and increase disability

Figure 1: Typical Journey of Health

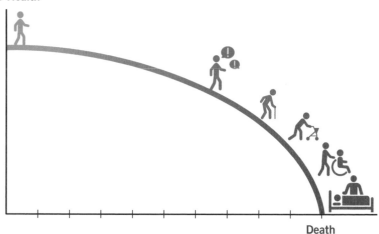

1. Make a Choice for Acceptable Quality of Life

Is your quality of life acceptable now? If yes, **Table 1** shows the treatment options. Choose a treatment now if you have an acceptable quality of life.

Table 1: Acceptable Quality of Life Treatment Options
The goal of treatment here may be to cure the illness and prolong life using every possible means.

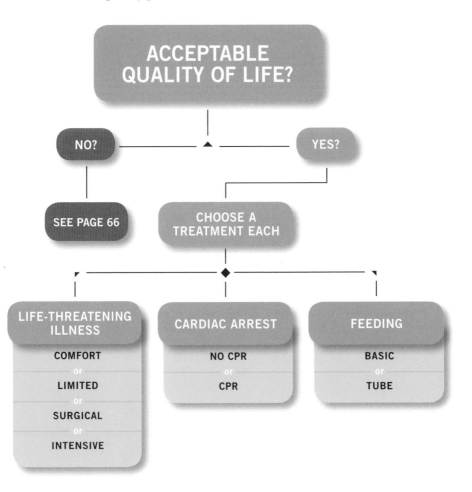

2. Make a choice for unacceptable quality of life that is irreversible

Figure 2 shows how disabilities can progress to a point where you might have a very poor or unacceptable quality of life.

What would you want if you are in a vegetative state or permanent coma – unable to communicate, move, swallow etc. and you need to be tube fed and will not recover because your condition is irreversible?

Figure 2: Progression of Disability from an Acceptable Quality of Life to an Unacceptable Quality of Life

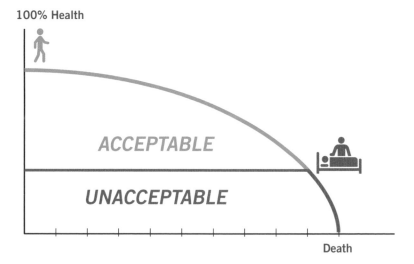

Consider a persistent vegetative state as the example of an unacceptable, severe disability. If you:

- Are in a Permanent Coma (persistent vegetative state)
- Are unable to recognise family
- Are unable to communicate basic needs
- Are unable to dress and groom
- Are unable to swallow
- Need to be tube fed
- Have no hope of recovery.

Now if you were in this condition, what choices would you make? Complete **Table 2** for an unacceptable quality of life.

Table 2: Unacceptable Quality of Life Treatment Options
Comfort measure only. The goal of treatment is not to prolong
life but to provide comfort at the end of life.

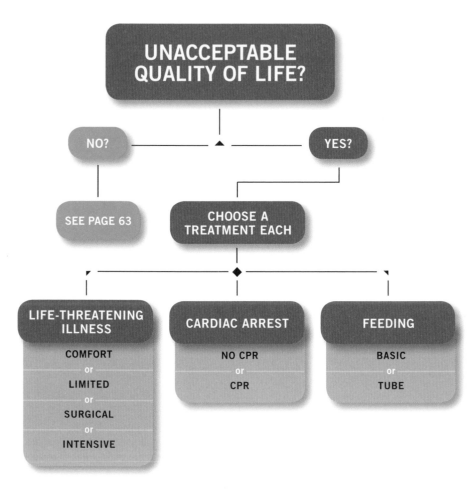

3. Making the Personal Statement

You have made your choices for an acceptable and unacceptable quality of life. Now it is time to make your personal statement. You have already established that a persistent vegetative state – permanent coma, is an unacceptable condition. Now you want to describe other conditions that you would consider intolerable. Use the list of conditions below. You can add others that you would consider unacceptable to the personal statement.

Would you consider these unacceptable/irreversible? **Yes** or **No**
- Permanent Coma
- Severe Dementia
- Incontinent of urine & stool because of confusion
- Unable to dress/groom because of confusion
- Unable to recognise family
- Unable to communicate basic needs
- Needs to be spoon fed
- Paralysed on one side
- Need to be lifted in and out of bed or chair
- Unable to walk alone
- Blind
- Deaf
- Incurable cancer i.e. cancer that has spread & cannot be cured.

Use these examples to complete the personal statement and include others you would consider unacceptable.

4. Choosing your proxy (designated decision maker)

Now you should decide who you want to be your proxy/power of attorney. If you become too ill to make your decision known –

who would you want to represent you? Contact the person or persons (if you want more than one) and discuss your choices. When you are happy you understand each other and go over your advance directive with your family doctor. Then together you can sign it and keep your own copies. You can then discuss how often you want to update it.

With whom should I discuss my Directive?

Discuss the directive with all those concerned before you complete it. Talk to your proxy, family, close friends and your doctor. Make sure the final decision is yours, and not the result of pressure from others. If your doctor disagrees with your decision, you may want to get a second opinion. You do not need a solicitor to complete this document. You may want to let your solicitor know you have an advance care directive when you are making out or updating a property will. You do not have to complete your advance care directive with your doctor, but it's a good idea to include your doctor because he may be called if you get sick. Your doctor is knowledgeable about health and personal issues and should be able to answer your questions. If your doctor knows what you want she can tell others what your wishes are when decisions need to be made.

How shall I store it?

Leave a copy with your doctor, your proxy and family. If you are admitted to a healthcare facility, the original form should go with you. Get photocopies and share them with your solicitor and family if you wish.

What if I change my mind?

Tell your proxy, your family and doctor. Update all the copies of the advance care directive every few years or if there is a change in your health. If you update and make no changes, just date and initial it with your doctor and proxy. If you make changes it is important to discuss these changes with your doctor and proxy and have them co-sign the updated documents.

Revoking the Advance Care Directive

To revoke this document, write down the revocation on paper, sign and date it, and have witnesses sign also. Notify your proxy, your family, your friends and family doctor and all those who were involved in preparing and signing the original document.

Updating the Directive

Decide how often you would like to review this document. For example, you may decide to review it once a year, or after any illness or change in your health. This decision will depend on your age, your health and life plans.

A sample of a completed advance care directive is provided for your consideration.

SAMPLE

LET ME DECIDE
THE ADVANCE CARE DIRECTIVE

Name of Adult:
Mary Browne

1. INTRODUCTION

In this Directive I, *Mary Browne* am stating my wishes for my health and personal care should the time ever come when I am not able to communicate because of illness or injury. This directive should never be used if I am able to decide for myself. It must never be substituted for my judgment, if I can make these decisions. If the time comes when I am unable to make these decisions, I would like this Directive to be followed and respected. Please do everything necessary to keep me comfortable and free of pain. Even though I may have indicated that I do not want certain treatments, I recognize that these may be necessary to keep me comfortable. I understand that my choices may be overridden if a treatment is necessary to maintain comfort. I have thought about and discussed my decision with my family, friends and my family doctor. In an emergency, please contact my Proxy Decision-Maker. If this person is not available, then please do as I have requested in this Directive.

2. PERSONAL STATEMENT

(Please refer to *Let Me Decide* for further guidance in completing this form.)

I would consider an unacceptable condition to be any condition:

1. *Where I was so confused that cannot recognize my family or communicate with my family.*

2. *Where others have to wash, dress and feed me.*

3. *If I was in a persistent vegetative state.*

4. *If I had incurable cancer that was causing me pain or other symptoms that could not be relieved.*

5. *Where I am permanently bed bound and others have to lift me in and out of bed*

6. *Where I can't communicate basic needs*

Signature: *Mary Browne*   Date: *17th June 2015*

Print Name: *MARY BROWNE*

I would agree to the following:	Yes	No
Blood Transfusion	☒	☐
Donating my organs to another after my death	☒	☐
Cremation	☒	☐

3. THE HEALTHCARE CHART

(One choice in each box below should be circled and written in the space underneath.)

If my condition is Reversible/Acceptable		
Life Threatening Illness	**Cardiac Arrest**	**Feeding**
Comfort Limited (Surgical) Intensive	No CPR (CPR)	Basic (Tubes)
Surgical	*CPR*	*Tubes*

If my condition is Irreversible/Intolerable		
Life Threatening Illness	**Cardiac Arrest**	**Feeding**
(Comfort) Limited Surgical Intensive	(No CPR) CPR	(Basic) Tubes
Comfort	*No CPR*	*Basic*

		Tom Browne,	
17 June 2015	*Mary Browne*	*Margaret Browne*	*Dr. Andrew Burke*
Date	Signature	Proxy Signature(s)	Physician Signature

Date of next review should be once a year, after an illness, or if there is any change in health

17 June 2016	Mary Browne	Tom Browne, Margaret Browne	Dr. Andrew Burke
Date	Signature	Proxy Signature(s)	Physician Signature

Date	Signature	Proxy Signature(s)	Physician Signature

4. DEFINITIONS

Levels of Care

Acceptable condition
Condition where I have an acceptable quality of life.

Intolerable (or unacceptable) condition
Condition where I have what I would consider to be an intolerable or unacceptable disability, and this is irreversible.

Feeding

Basic
- Spoon feed with regular diet
- Give all food and fluids by mouth that can be tolerated
- Give supplements or special diets (e.g. high calorie, fat or protein supplements) if needed.

Tubes
People who can't eat can be fed by tubes passed into the stomach (stomach tubes) or by giving food directly into the blood (intravenous tube).
(a) Intravenous
(b) Stomach

(a) Intravenous
Give nutrients (water, salt, carbohydrate, protein and fat) by intravenous infusions directly into the veins. This is called Total Parenteral Nutrition.

(b) Stomach Tubes
Into the stomach. There are two main types.
Nasogastric Tube: a soft plastic tube passed through the nose or mouth into the stomach.

Gastrostomy Tube: a soft plastic tube passed directly into the stomach through the skin over the abdomen.

Cardiac Arrest, Cardio-Pulmonary Resuscitation (CPR)

No CPR

Make no attempt to resuscitate. (No cardiac massage, electrical shock(s) to the heart or artificial/mechanical breathing support)

CPR

Use cardiac massage and artificial/mechanical breathing. May include placement of tubes in the throat to the lungs (endotracheal tubes), electric shock to the chest and heart (defibrillation), intravenous fluids and drugs. CPR may result in damage to ribs (fractures) and/or lungs as a result of mechanical/artificial ventilation and chest compressions.

Treatment of Life-Threatening Illness:

Comfort or Palliative Care
- Keep me warm, dry and pain free
- Do not transfer to hospital unless absolutely necessary
- Only give measures that enhance comfort or minimize pain
- Intravenous line started only if it improves comfort
- No x-rays, blood tests or antibiotics unless they are given to improve comfort.

Limited Care (includes Comfort or Palliative Care)
- May or may not transfer to hospital
- Intravenous therapy may be appropriate
- A trial of appropriate drugs, like antibiotics, may be used
- No invasive procedures
- Do not transfer to Intensive Care Unit (ICU).

Surgical Care (includes Limited Care)
- Transfer to acute care hospital (where patient may be evaluated)
- Emergency surgery if necessary
- Do not admit to Intensive Care Unit (ICU)
- Do not ventilate (except during and after surgery i.e. tube down throat and connected to a machine)
- Includes Kidney Dialysis.

Intensive Care (includes Surgical Care)
- Transfer to acute care hospital without hesitation
- Admit to Intensive Care Unit (ICU) if necessary
- Ventilate if necessary
- Insert central line (i.e. main arteries for fluids when other veins collapse
- Provide surgery, biopsies, all life-support systems and transplant surgery
- Do everything possible to maintain life.

DONOR (Person Completing The Directive)

Signature: *Mary Browne*

Date: *17 June 2017*

Print Name: *MARY BROWNE*

Tel. (H): *(021) 420-0001*

Tel. (W): *(021) 420-0002*

Mobile Tel.: *(086) 420-0003*

Address: *1234 High Street, Dublin*

5. PROXY (Over 18 Years Of Age)

Signature: *Tom Browne*

Date: *17 June 2017*

Print Name: *TOM BROWNE*

Tel. (H): *(021) 420-0001*

Tel. (W): *(021) 420-0002*

Mobile Tel.: *(086) 420-0004*

Address: *1234 High Street, Dublin*

ALTERNATE PROXY (Over 18 Years Of Age)

Signature: *Margaret Browne*

Date: *17 June 2017*

Print Name: *MARGARET BROWNE*

Tel. (H): *(021) 420-0005*

Tel. (W): *(021) 420-0006*

Mobile Tel.: *(086) 420-0007*

Address: *9876 College Rd, Dublin*

WITNESS SIGNATURE

I am witness to this Healthcare Directive, I have signed in the presence of the person who has completed this directive. I am not a close family member of either the Donor or the Proxy. I do not expect to receive any financial benefit from the estate of the Donor. I have no reason to believe that the Donor is incapable of understanding or giving these instructions. I am over 18 years of age.

Signature: *Karen Smith*

Date: *17 June 2017*

Print Name: *KAREN SMITH*

Tel. (H): *(021) 111-0008*   Tel. (W): *(021) 111-4444*

Mobile Tel.: *(086) 420-0010*

Address: *1234 Western Road, Dublin*

Signature: *John Murphy*

Date: *17 June 2017*

Print Name: *JOHN MURPHY*

Tel. (H): *(021) 111-0008*   Tel. (W): *(021) 111-4444*

Mobile Tel.: *(086) 420-0010*

Address: *1234 Western Road, Dublin*

FAMILY PHYSICIAN

Signature: *Dr. Andrew Burke*

Date: *17 June 2017*

Print Name: *DR. ANDREW BURKE*

Tel. (H): *(021) 420-0011*

Tel. (W): *(021) 420-0012*

Mobile Tel.: *(086) 420-0013*

Address: *5678 Grand Parade, Dublin*

GLOSSARY OF TERMS

Advance Care Directive: An advance care directive is a document that people fill out in advance when they are capable to let others know what healthcare they would want if they become incapable later. Healthcare providers may not act directly on an Advance Care Directive – they must consult with an appropriate Proxy where possible. The Advance Care Directive however may assist in directing the Proxy. It is also known as a Living Will or Instructional Directive. The *Let Me Decide* Advance Care Directive has an instructional and proxy directive. This provides double reinforcement that your wishes are followed. If your proxy is not available during a crisis, the written instructions in the instructional part informs healthcare providers of your wishes. The instructional part, clearly lays out what you would want for a whole variety of eventualities.

Advance Directive: An advance directive is a written statement that expresses a person's wishes in advance. The most widely used advance directive is a Will. It contains instructions to inform others how you want your possessions distributed after death.

Aids: Acquired Immune Deficiency Syndrome has been strongly linked to the Human Immunodeficiency Virus (HIV), which weakens the body's defence against disease. It is transmitted by the exchange of certain specific body fluids under specific circumstances, and not by casual contact. There is no known cure.

Alzheimer's Disease: A disease of the brain causing progressive memory loss. With time, there is loss of ability to learn and, eventually, loss of the ability to do even simple tasks. The patient's behaviour may also change. There is no known cure.

Anaesthetic: A local anaesthetic 'freezes' the skin by making it numb to pain. With general anaesthetic, a person is temporarily 'put to sleep': this is used only for major medical procedures.

Angina or Angina Pectoris: Chest pain due to poor blood-flow to the heart, which usually occurs with exercise, and goes away with rest. The pain may spread to the arms and/or neck. This means that the blood supply to the heart is inadequate. If it persists, the heart muscle may be damaged and result in a heart attack.

Antibiotics: Drugs used to treat infections caused by bacteria.

Basic Life Support: Mouth-to-mouth resuscitation and heart massage (see CPR, below).

Best Interest: This term is usually used in reference to a decision made on behalf of another individual that accounts for the needs and welfare of that individual. For example, the decision a parent makes for their child is normally made in the child's best interest. It differs from a 'substitute decision' which is one that closely approximates the decision the individual would have made for himself or herself. If you were told what a person wanted then you would do the same thing exactly. If you did not know what a person wanted then you would ask yourself, *"What would he/ she have done based on what I know of their values and previous track record."* In this case, you are making decisions that you think the person would have made and acting in their Best Interest. Best Interest is when you don't know exactly what the person would want and you are guessing what you think what decision/choice that person would have wanted based on your knowledge of the person in the past.

Biopsy: Surgical removal of tissue so that it may be examined under a microscope for evidence of disease.

Blood Transfusion: The injection of a volume of blood, previously taken from a healthy person, into a patient, i.e. where blood from one person is given to another.

Bronchoscopy: A procedure in which the physician looks through a flexible tube into the airways of the lungs, using a scope with a light on the tip.

Bypass Surgery: Replacement or re-routing of blood vessels to an area of the body where the blood flow is not adequate.

Cardiac Arrest: Stoppage of heartbeat.

Cardio-Pulmonary Resuscitation (CPR): Is an emergency procedure that attempts to restore breathing and heartbeat in a person whose heart or breathing, or both, have stopped. CPR involves external cardiac massage (pumping on the chest to push the blood through the heart) and mouth-to-mouth breathing. It may also include drugs, electric defibrillators (machines to shock the heart into action) or a breathing machine (mechanical ventilation).

CHF: Congestive Heart Failure, caused by failure of the heart to maintain adequate circulation of blood, resulting in weakness and shortness of breath.

Chronic Bronchitis: Severe inflammation of the mucous membrane in the bronchial tubes (conducting air from the mouth to the lungs).

Colonoscopy: A procedure in which a physician looks into the large bowel through a flexible tube known as a scope.

Comfort Care: (Treatment choice for life threatening illness): This is a treatment option for life threatening illness in the *Let Me Decide* Directive, this level of care provides comfort and relief from pain and other symptoms, but does not aim to cure a condition. Elements of the Palliative Care Approach & Palliative Care can apply to comfort care (See definitions below).

Conditions/Disability – Intolerable/Irreversible/Unacceptable: Condition/medical treatments where you have what you would consider to be an intolerable or unacceptable disability, and this is irreversible.

Conditions/Disability – Reversible/Acceptable: Condition/medical treatments where you have an acceptable quality of life.

COPD: Chronic Obstructive Pulmonary Disease, caused by problems in the airways leading to the lungs or in the lungs themselves. The main symptom is chronic shortness of breath.

Cornea: The clear, front surface of the eye.

Corneal Transplant: Surgical replacement of a damaged cornea with a donated cornea.

CPR: Cardio-Pulmonary Resuscitation, the use of mouth-to-mouth breathing and heart massage to restore heartbeat.

Cremation: To consume (a corpse etc.) by extreme heat/fire in a furnace. It takes place at a crematorium. Cremation is an alternative to burial when someone dies. Most Christian denominations and other religious sects around the world permit cremation.

CT: Computerized Tomography or CAT scan, use of a computer to produce, from x-ray data, a view of part of the body.

Cystic Fibrosis: An inherited disease that causes chronic lung infections and poor function of the pancreas in young people. There is no known cure, but treatment can prolong the patient's life to about 30 years of age.

Decisional Capacity: The ability of adults to give valid consent. They are able to understand the information provided to them about their health condition as well as alternatives and options for treatment and able to deliberate on the particular choices in terms of their own personal values and preferences, make a decision, and communicate that decision.

Defibrillator: An instrument that shocks the heart with an electric current to revive it or to correct its rhythm.

Definitions: Section in the *Let Me Decide* Advance Care Directive which contains explanations of terms used in the Directive.

Dehydration: Loss of water from the body. Is where fluids are lost from the body (dry skin, dry mouth) and people experience thirst.

Dialysis: A method of filtering and cleaning the blood of patients with kidney problems.

Donor: Person who is completing the Advance Care Directive and nominating a Proxy.

ECG: Electrocardiogram. A record of the heartbeat traced by an electrocardiograph. An instrument recording the electrical currents generated (non-invasively) by a person's heartbeat. Tracing of the electrical function of the heart.

ECT: Electroconvulsive Therapy, the use of an electric shock to treat specific types of mental illness, for example, acute depression.

EEG: Electroencephalogram, a method of measuring brain activity.

EMG: Electromyelogram, a method of measuring muscle and nerve function.

Endoscopy: Looking inside any body cavity by means of a scope.

External Cardiac Massage: Massage of the heart by applying pressure on the chest to maintain circulation.

Feeding – Basic: At this level of care you would receive a regular diet (fluids and solids).

Feeding – Gastrostomy Tube: A surgical opening in the abdominal wall so that a tube can be put directly into the stomach, usually for feeding. (See also Stomach Tubes and Nasogastric Tubes).

Feeding – Intravenous (IV): At this level, fluids can be given directly into the veins. The needles required for intravenous feeding eventually damage the veins. Intravenous lines can be inserted into the large veins near the heart, using minor procedures under local anaesthetic. This method of feeding is called Total Parenteral Nutrition.

Feeding – Nasogastric Tube: Tubes put down the nose and into the stomach for feeding or drainage. (See also Stomach Tubes and Gastrostomy Tubes).

Feeding – Stomach Tubes: See also Nasogastric Tubes and Gastrostomy Tubes.

Feeding – Subcutaneous: To maintain hydration, fluids can be given directly into the veins via intravenous lines. Fluids can also be given through tiny plastic tubes placed just under the skin (subcutaneous), usually on the abdomen. These needles need to be changed every few days. It is not possible to feed people through subcutaneous tubes.

Feeding – Total Parenteral Nutrition: Complete nutrition (proteins, sugars, fats, vitamins and minerals) given by injection through a vein. (See also Intravenous (IV) Feeding).

Fibre-Optic Scope: An instrument used for looking inside body cavities.

Fractured Hip: A break in the thigh bone (the femur) between the hip and the knee. Breaks usually occur at the upper part of the femur just below the hip bone (the pelvis).

Healthcare: Anything that is done for a therapeutic, preventive, palliative, cosmetic or other purpose related to health.

Healthcare Chart: Section in the *Let Me Decide* Advance Care Directive where people state their wishes for treatment of life-threatening illness, cardiac arrest and feeding, depending on whether your condition is acceptable or unacceptable.

Healthcare Provider: A person who (under a prescribed act) is licensed, certified or registered to provide healthcare.

Hepatitis: Swelling of the liver, caused by alcohol abuse, viral, or bacterial infections.

Hydration: Also known as Rehydration is where fluids are given to restore the normal fluid balance.

ICU: Intensive Care Unit is a specialized department in a hospital that provides intensive care medicine (Medical treatment with constant monitoring etc. of a seriously ill patient). Also known as critical care unit (CCU), intensive therapy unit, or intensive treatment unit (ITU). Many hospitals also have designated intensive care areas for certain specialties of medicine, depending on the needs and resources of the hospital.

IHD: Ischemic Heart Disease. Also known as Ischemic or myocardial ischemia, is a disease characterized by ischemia (reduced blood supply) of the heart muscle, usually due to narrowing of the arteries in the heart, and is called coronary artery disease (atherosclerosis of the coronary arteries). Risk increases with age, smoking, hypercholesterolemia (high cholesterol levels), diabetes, and hypertension (high blood pressure), and is more common in men and those who have close relatives with ischemic heart disease.

Incontinence: Loss of control of bladder or bowel.

Instructional Directive: An instructional directive states which treatments are wanted or not wanted under any given circumstance. These statements can be general or specific. The more specific the instructions, the easier it will be for family and doctors to follow. Instructional directives are also called Living Wills. An instructional directive is not limited to the treatment of terminal or irreversible conditions – it can also apply to curable, reversible conditions. If your proxy is not available during a crisis, the written instructions in the instructional part informs healthcare providers of your wishes. The instructional part, clearly lays out what you would want for a whole variety of eventualities.

Intensive Care (Treatment choice for life threatening illness): This is a treatment option for life threatening illness in the Let Me Decide Directive. At this level of care everything a modern hospital has to offer would be used to maintain your life. You would receive surgery, biopsies and life-support systems (kidney machines, breathing machines). Some patients might receive transplant surgery if necessary (including heart, kidney, liver or bone-marrow transplants). If you were at home, you would be transferred to hospital. If you were in a small community hospital, you could be transferred to a larger hospital for a wider range of diagnostic tests and treatments. It is important to remember that just because you request intensive care – you might not necessarily receive it – either because you do not require it, would not benefit from it, or it is not available. You will not automatically receive your chosen level of care for every illness. For example, if you asked for intensive care for a life-threatening illness, you would not automatically be admitted to intensive care every time you became ill. If admitted to hospital with a bleeding ulcer, for example, you might not necessarily require intensive care. Intensive care will only be provided, if beds are available and your condition meets the criteria for admission set out by the unit. On the other hand, if you requested comfort/palliative care for an illness, you might have surgery. If you broke your hip and had severe pain, surgery might be the only way to relieve your pain. In this case you could receive surgery to put a pin and plate in the bone to fix the hip and relieve the pain. In this case, surgery is performed to relieve suffering and keep you comfortable. It is not given to prolong your life but to relieve pain. In this case surgery may be considered part of 'comfort/palliative' care.

Intestine: Bowel.

Intolerable/Unacceptable: Disability that is associated with such a poor quality of life that the person would not want technology used to prolong life. At this stage the person would just want comfort/palliative care for life threatening illness and No CPR in the event of cardiac arrest.

Intravenous (IV): Injection of fluids into the body through a fine tube into a vein.

Introduction: Section in the *Let Me Decide* Advance Care Directive where people state the reasons why they want to complete the directive. It advises others that the directive should not be used while you are capable of making decisions for yourself. It should only be used if you are incapacitated by disease or injury and unable to make your own decisions. It revokes previous documents and establishes this document as the latest expression of your wishes.

Investigations: Tests done by the doctor, such as blood tests, scans, x-rays, etc.

Irreversible Illness: An illness that cannot be cured.

Kidney Machine: The machine used in dialysis to clean the blood of people with kidney problems.

Laparoscopy: A fibre-optic tube passed through the abdominal wall to give a view of the organs in the abdomen.

Laparotomy: Surgery to explore the abdomen, usually to find the cause of pain or blockage.

Life Support: Machines used to keep a person alive by maintaining circulation and ventilation (breathing).

Life-Threatening Illness: Any illness that can cause death.

Limited Care: (Treatment choice for life threatening illness): This is a treatment option for life threatening illness in the *Let Me Decide* Directive, this level of care includes more treatment than 'comfort/supportive', but less than 'surgical'. For example, if you wanted limited care and developed pneumonia, you could receive antibiotics, blood tests, intravenous fluids, x-rays and oxygen. If you had bleeding from the stomach or intestine, you could receive blood transfusions and drugs to stop the bleeding. You would not receive emergency surgery to stop the bleeding or medical tests that required a general anaesthetic. You would not be put on life-support machines. You would not go on a kidney machine (for dialysis) if your kidneys failed. If you were at home when you became ill, you could be transferred to hospital if enough care could not be provided at home.

Living Will: See Advance Care Directive and Instructional Directive above.

Major Healthcare: Healthcare including, for example, major surgery, a general anaesthetic, major diagnostic or investigative procedures, radiation therapy, intravenous chemotherapy, kidney dialysis, Electroconvulsive Therapy (ECT) and laser surgery.

Minor Healthcare: Any treatment that is not major healthcare. For example, immunizations, blood tests, routine dental fillings and extractions, and routine clinical procedures such as suturing of a cut or wound.

Naming Others: Section in the *Let Me Decide* Advance Care Directive which contains the names, addresses and telephone numbers of your family doctor, proxy(s) and witnesses. Home and work numbers are given, along with additional numbers where these people can be reached in an emergency.

Near Relative: A spouse, adult child, parent, adult brother or sister or other adult relation by birth or adoption.

No CPR (Cardio-Pulmonary Resuscitation) Order: This order means that no attempt will be made to revive a person whose breathing or heart, or both, have stopped.

Organ Donation: Where a person agrees to give their organs to another after death.

Palliative Care (Treatment choice for life threatening illness): This is a treatment option for life threatening illness in the *Let Me Decide* Directive, this level of care provides comfort and relief.

Palliative Care: Palliative care is an approach that improves the quality of life of persons and their families facing the problems associated with life-threatening illness, through the prevention and relief of suffering by means of early identification and impeccable assessment and treatment of pain and other problems, physical, psychosocial and spiritual.

Palliative care:
- Provides relief from pain and other distressing symptoms
- Affirms life and regards dying as a normal process
- Intends neither to hasten or postpone death
- Integrates the psychological and spiritual aspects of patient care
- Offers a support system to help persons live as actively as possible until death
- Offers a support system to help the family cope during the patients illness and in their own bereavement
- Uses a team approach to address the needs of persons and their families, including bereavement counselling, if indicated

- Will enhance quality of life, and may also positively influence the course of illness
- Is applicable early in the course of illness, in conjunction with other therapies that are intended to prolong life, such as chemotherapy or radiation therapy, and includes those investigations needed to better understand and manage distressing clinical complications.

Palliative Care Approach: The palliative care approach aims to promote both physical and psychosocial well-being. It is a vital and integral part of all clinical practice, whatever the illness or its stage, informed by a knowledge and practice of palliative care principles.

Paraplegia: Loss of all sensation and movement in the lower half of the body.

Parkinson's Disease: A disorder of part of the brain, causing a tremor ('shakes') when at rest, difficulty rising from chairs, and a slow, shuffling walk. Although not curable, symptoms can be improved with medication.

Persistent Vegetative State: Permanent Coma, unable to communicate or swallow or more. This person needs to be tube fed.

Personal Care Issues: Section in the *Let Me Decide* Advance Care Directive where people state where they want to reside, nutritional needs, personal safety issues, clothing and hygiene needs.

Personal Statement: Section in the *Let Me Decide* Advance Care Directive where people state what level of irreversible disability they consider unacceptable, and express their wishes regarding levels of care, post mortem, organ donation, blood transfusion, and cremation or burial.

Pneumonia: Infection and congestion of the lungs.

Post Mortem: Autopsy, usually to find the cause of death.

Prostate Cancer: Cancer of prostate gland in males.

Proxy: An adult that substitutes for another adult Donor (person completing the Advance Care Directive). This is a substitute decision maker. A proxy would be expected to make the same decision as the adult Donor for whom they are acting.

Proxy Directive: A proxy is a substitute or power of attorney who you (the donor) nominate to make decisions for you if you become incapable. The person who is completing the advance care directive is called the donor. A proxy directive is the document the donor completes to name another to make decisions for his/her health or personal care if he/she becomes incapable. This proxy has the ability to make health and personal care decisions in much the same way as a financial power of attorney can manage finances. If your proxy is not available during a crisis, the written instructions in the instructional part informs healthcare providers of your wishes. The instructional part, clearly lays out what you would want for a whole variety of eventualities.

Pulmonary Embolism: Blood clot in the lung that often arises or breaks off from a clot in the calves.

Quadriplegia: Loss of all sensation and movement below the neck.

Rehydration: Also known as Hydration is where fluids are given to restore the normal fluid balance.

Resuscitate: To restore life by giving mouth-to-mouth breathing and/or heart massage.

Reversible Illness: An illness that can be cured.

Scan: A method of looking inside the body without surgery can involve the injection of a dye that can be seen by a special x-ray.

SLE: Systemic Lupus Erythematosus (Lupus), a chronic disease that affects many organs, joints and skin. It is caused when the body's defence mechanism turns on itself. The course of the disease varies greatly from person to person; however, it is not curable.

Special Diet: Diet geared to the specific nutritional needs of patients with medical conditions such as diabetes, coeliac, cholesterol; personal lifestyle e.g. vegetarian, and also religious dietary needs.

Spouse: A person who either is married to another person and is not living separate and apart, or is living with another person in a marriage-like relationship (including a same sex relationship).

Stroke: Sudden damage to the brain caused by lack of oxygen, often resulting in weakness, slurred speech, loss of movement, etc. These losses may or may not improve over time.

Surgical Care (Treatment choice for life threatening illness):
This is a treatment option for life threatening illness in the *Let Me Decide* Directive, at this level of care you would receive all the measures included in 'limited' care, like blood tests, x-rays, but in addition you could have surgery, and be put on a kidney machine, if necessary. You would be put on a breathing machine (ventilator) during or after surgery, if necessary. Some people need ventilators for a short time after surgery until they are able to breathe on their own again. You would receive intravenous fluids and blood transfusions if you had life-threatening bleeding. A tube might be passed into the bowel (endoscopy) to find the cause of bleeding. If necessary, doctors would perform surgery to stop the source of the bleeding. You would not be transferred to intensive care, unless that was necessary to keep you comfortable. You would be transferred from home to hospital, without hesitation, for surgical care, if it was necessary.

Supportive Care (Treatment choice for life threatening illness):
This is a treatment option for life threatening illness in the *Let Me Decide* Directive, this level of care provides comfort and relief from pain and other symptoms, but does not aim to cure a condition. Elements of the Palliative Care Approach & Palliative Care can apply to supportive care (See definitions above).

Terminal Illness: Illness from which a person will not recover and will die within hours or days from an incurable life limiting illness.

Threshold: A certain point at which a disability may become intolerable/unacceptable.

TIA: Transient Ischemic Attack, temporary block of the blood supply to the brain, causing weakness, slurred speech, loss of movement and memory lapses, lasting from a few moments to several hours.

Transplant: An organ or tissue taken from the body for use in another area of the same body or for use in another person's body.

Urgent/Emergency Healthcare: Healthcare that must be provided without delay to prevent harm or death. Consent is not required if it cannot be obtained from the donor, although if the donor's Proxy is available and authorized to make the decision, the healthcare provider should act in accordance with the decision of the Proxy.

Ventilator: Breathing machine or respirator.

Will: A document that contains instructions to inform others how you want your possessions distributed after death. (See also Advance Directives above).

Witness: A person who co-signs the *Let Me Decide* Advance Care Directive. A witness can be anyone except a close family member, anyone who might expect a financial benefit from the estate, the Proxy(s), the Proxy(s) spouse or children (natural or adopted) or anyone who is under 18 years of age.

LET ME DECIDE PUBLICATIONS

1. Clarnette, R.M. & Molloy, D.W. Healthcare directives: The Annual of Medical Direction 1991: 48-51.

2. Molloy, D.W., Guyatt, G.H., Alemayehu, E. & McIlroy, W.E. Treatment preferences, attitudes towards advance directives and concerns about healthcare. Humane Medicine 1991; 7: 285-290.

3. Molloy, D.W. & Guyatt, G.H. A comprehensive healthcare directive in a home for the aged. Can Med Assoc J 1991; 145: 307-311.

4. Alemayehu, E., Molloy, D.W., Guyatt, G.H. et al. Variability in physicians' decisions on caring for chronically ill elderly patients: an international study. Can Med Assoc J 1991; 144: 1133-1138.

5. Molloy, D.W., Guyatt, G.H., Alemayehu, E. et. al. Factors affecting physicians' decisions on caring for an incompetent elderly patient: an international study. Canada Med Assoc J 1991; 145: 947-952.

6. Molloy, D.W., Clarnette, R., Braun, E.A. et al. Decision making in the incompetent elderly: the daughter from California syndrome. J Am Geriatric Soc 1991; 39: 336-339.

7. Lever, J.A., Molloy, D.W., Eisemann, M. et al. Variability in nurses' decisions about the care of chronically ill elderly – an international study. Humane Medicine 1992; 8: 138-144.

8. Molloy, D.W., Urbanyi, M., Horsman, J.R., Guyatt, G.H. & Bédard, M. Two years experience with a comprehensive healthcare directive in a home for the aged. Annals RCPSC 1992; 25: 433-436.

9. Urbanyi, M., Molloy, D.W. & Lever, J.A. Healthcare directives for the elderly. Can Fam Physician 1992; 38: 2357-2361.

10. Molloy, D.W., Harrison, C., Farrugia, M.C. & Cunje, A. The Canadian experience with advance treatment directives.
Humane Medicine 1993; 1: 70-77.

11. Darzins, P.J., Molloy, D.W. & Harrison, C.N. Treatment for life-threatening illness. N Engl J Med Sept 1993; 2: 736.

12. Molloy, W.D., Guyatt, G., Alemayehu, E., McIroy, W. (1993), Treatment Preferences Attitudes Toward Advance Directives and Concerns About Healthcare, New England Journal of Medicine, pp. 736

13. Gordan, G., Mitchell, A., Molloy, W.D., Capretta, R., Horsman, J., Griffith, L. (1994) Measuring Patient and Relative Satisfaction with Level of Aggressiveness of Care and Involvement in Care Decisions in the Context of Life Threatening Illness, Journal of Clinical Epidemiology, pp. 1215 – 1224

14. Harrison, C., Molloy, D.W., Darzins, P.J. & Bédard, M. Should people do unto others as they would not want done unto themselves? J Clinical Ethics1995; 6: 1419

15. Cook, D.J., Guyatt, G.H., Jaeschke, R. et al. Determinants in Canadian healthcare workers of the decision to withdraw life support from the critically ill. JAMA 1995; 273: 703-708.

16. Guyatt, G.H., Mitchell, A., Molloy, D.W. et al. Measuring patient and relative satisfaction with level of aggressiveness and care and involvement in care decisions in the context of life threatening illness. J Clin. Epidemiol 1995; 48; 1215-1224.

17. Molloy, D.W., Silberfeld, M., Darzins, P.J. et al. Measuring capacity to complete an advance healthcare directive. J Am Geriatric Soc 1996; 44: 660-664.

18. James, J., Molloy, D.W., Urbanyi, M. & Rapelje, D.H. The right to die with dignity. Canadian Healthcare Management June 1996; 78-82.

19. Molloy, D.W., Jubelius, R. & Parish S. Implementing advance directives across care sectors. Canadian Healthcare Management. November 1996; 143-146.

20. Molloy, D.W., Bédard, M., Guyatt, G.H. et al. Attitudes, training issues and barriers for community nurses implementing an advance directive program Perspectives, 1997; 21: 2-8.

21. Patterson, C., Molloy, D.W., Jubelius, R., Guyatt, G.H. & Bédard, M. Provisional educational needs of healthcare providers in palliative care in three nursing homes in Ontario. Journal of Palliative Care 1997; 13: 3; 13-17.

22. Molloy, D.W., Guyatt, G.H., Goeree, R. et al. A comprehensive healthcare directive for competent and incompetent residents of a home for the aged. Annals RCPSC 1997; 30: 339-345.

23. Patterson, C., Molloy, D.W., Guyatt, G.H. et al. Systematic implementation of an advance healthcare directive in the community. Canadian Journal of Nursing Administration 1997; 10: 96-108.

24. Molloy, D.W. Advance directives in long term care facilities. Long Term Care February/March 1998; 8: 2-3.

25. Strang, D., Molloy, D.W. & Harrison, C. Capacity to choose place of residence: autonomy vs. beneficence. J of Palliative Care 1998; 14: 25-29.

26. Molloy, D.W., Jubelius, R. & Darzins, P.J. Competency To Complete an Advance Directive. Capacity to Decide Book, Chapter 8, Newgrange Press August 1998.

27. Eisemann, M., Richter, J., Bauer, B., Bonelli, R. & Porzsolt, F. Physicians' decision-making in incompetent elderly patients: a comparative study between Austria, Germany (East, West) and Sweden. Int. Psychogeriatr. 1999; 11: 313-324.

28. Molloy, D.W., Russo, R., Pedlar, D. & Bédard, M. Implementation of advance directives among community-dwelling veterans. The Gerontologist 2000; 40: 213-217.

29. Molloy, D.W., Guyatt, G.H., Russo, R. et al. Systematic Implementation of an advance directive program in nursing homes: a randomized controlled trial. JAMA; 2000: 283; 1437-1442.

30. Molloy, D.W., Stiller, A. & Russo, R. Technology and educating seniors about advance directives. Educational Gerontologist 2000

31. Molloy, D.W., Russo, R., Stiller, A., Smith, S. & O'Donnell, 2000 "How to Implement the *Let me Decide* Advance Health and Personal Care Programme" JCOM Vol.

32. Vertesi, A., Lever, J., Molloy, D.W., Sanderson, B.,Tuttle, I.,Pokoradi, L., Principi, E., (2001) Standardized Mini Mental State Examination, Canadian Family Physician.

33. Stiller, A., Molloy, W., Russo, R., Dubois, S., Kavsak, Bedard, M (2001), "Development and Evaluation New Instrument to Implement Advance Directives", JCOM, Vol 8 (4).

34. Caplan, G.A., Meller, A., Squires, B., Chan, S., Willett, W., Advance care planning and hospital in the nursing home. Age and Ageing 2006; 35: 581-585 doi:10.1093/ageing/afl063 28 June 2006

35. McGlade, C., Molloy, D.W., Timmons, S., Decision-making in incompetent older adults: Clinical, Social and Legal issues. Medico-legal Journal of Ireland, 2011. 17(2):p70-75

36. Coffey, A., McCarthy, G., Weathers, E., Friedman, M. Isabel; Gallo, K., Ehrenfeld, M., Itzhaki, M., Chan, S., Li, W., Poletti, P., Zanotti, R., Molloy, D.W, McGlade, C., Fitzpatrick, J. 2013. Nurses' preferred end-of-life treatment choices in five countries. International Nursing Review, 2013. 60(3): 313-9. doi: 10.1111/inr.12024

37. Coffey, A., McCarthy, G., Weathers, E., Friedman, M. Isabel; Gallo, K., Ehrenfeld, M., Itzhaki, M., Chan, S., Li, W., Poletti, P., Zanotti, R., Molloy, D.W, McGlade, C., Fitzpatrick, J. 2013. Nurses' preferred end-of-life treatment choices in five countries. International Nursing Review, 2013. 60(3): 313-9. doi:10.1111/inr.12024

38. Sweeney, C., Molloy, DW., O'Caoimh, R., Bond, R., Hynes, H., McGlade,. C, Shorten, G., European Innovation Partnership on Active and Healthy Ageing: Ireland and the COL-LAGE experience. Irish Journal of Medical Science, 2013.182; S(6):p278-279.

39. O'Caoimh, R., Cornally, N., O'Herlihy, E., Gao, Y., Cronin, U., Coveney, S., Clarnette, R., McGlade, C., Molloy, DW., Opinions towards a consensus on Use of Medications in Advanced Dementia. Irish Journal of Medical Science, 2014. 183;S(7):p312

40. Coveney, S., Cornally, N., Coffey, A., McGlade, C., Daly, E., O'Caoimh, R., Molloy, DW., Too Much, Too Late: Polypharmacy at End-of-Life. Irish Journal of Medical Science, 2014. 183; S (7):p331.

41. Cornally, N., McGlade, C., Weathers, E., Daly, E., Fitzgerald, C., O'Caoimh, R., Coffey, A., Molloy, DW., Evaluating the systematic implementation of the Let me Decide advance care planning programme in long term care through focus groups: A user's perspective. BMC Palliative Care 2015. Published DOI 10.1186/s12904-015-0051-x

42. Coffey,. A, Weathers, E., McGlade, C., O'Caoimh, R., Daly, E., Svendrovski,A., McLoughlin, K., Molloy, DW., Measuring Staff Perception of End-of-Life Experience of Older Adults in Long Term Care. Applied Nursing Research, 2015 Published doi:10.1016/j.apnr.2015.05.

43. O'Caoimh, R., Sweeney, C., Hynes, H., McGlade, C., Cornally, N., Daly, E., Weathers, E., Coffey, A., Fitzgerald. C., O'Herlihy, E., Healy, E., O'Connell, E., O'Keeffe, G., Timmons, S., Foley, T., Creed, E., Hynes, M., Twomey, A., Sammon, M., Cullen, D., Mullan, E., Orfila, F., Paul, C., Clarnette, R., Campbell, S., Lupari, M., McCarthy, S., Sahm, L., Byrne, S., O'Leary, C., O'Shea, S., O'Donoghue, J., McAdoo, J., Kearney, P., Galvin, P., O'Byrne-Maguire, I.,, Brown J., Kenny, R., McFarlane, A., Deery, M., Bond, R., Molloy, D.W., Martin, J., Shorten, G., Collaboration on AGEing-COLLAGE: Ireland's Three Star Reference site for the European Innovation Partnership on Active and Healthy Ageing (EIP on AHA). European Geriatric Medicine,2015.6(5):505-511 doi:http://dx.doi.org/10/1016/j.eurger.2015.04.009

44. Daly, E., McGlade, C., Cornally, N., Weathers, E., O'Caoimh, R., McCarthy, J., Cronin U., Molloy, D.W., Challenges in implementing an advance care planning programme in long-term care. Journal of Nursing Ethics, 2015 DOI: 10.1186/s 12904-015-0051-x

45. O'Sullivan, R., Murphy, A., O'Caoimh, R., Cornally, N., Svendrovski, A., Daly, B., Fitzgerald, C., Twomey, C., McGlade, C., Molloy, D.W., Title: Economic Analysis of Systematically Implementing a Programme of Advance Care Planning in Three Irish Nursing Homes. Journal: BMC Research Notes DOI:10.1186/s13104-016-2048-9

46. Coffey, A., McCarthy, G., Weathers, E., Friedman, M. I., Gallo, K., Ehrenfeld, M., Chan, S., Li, W. H. C., Poletti, P., Zanotti, R., Molloy, D. W., McGlade, C., Fitzpatrick, J. J., and Itzhaki, M. (2016) Nurses' knowledge of advance directives and perceived confidence in end of life care: a cross ¬sectional study in five countries. International Journal of Nursing Practice, doi: 10.1111/ijn.12417 International Journal of Nursing Practice – IJNP-2014-00506.R2 Published on line: 28 Jan 2016.
Cornally, N., Coffey, A., Daly, E., McGlade, C., Weathers, E., O'Herlihy, E., O'Caoimh, R., McLoughlin, K., Svendrovski, A., and Molloy, W., 2016. Measuring staff perception of end of life experience of older adults in long term care. Applied Nursing Research 201630; p.245-251. doi:http://dx.doi.org/10.2016j.apnr.2015.05.015

47. Weathers, E., O'Caoimh, R., Cornally, N., Fitzgerald,C., Kearns, T., Coffey, A., Daly, E., O'Sullivan, R., McGlade, C., Molloy, DW., Advance care planning: A systemic review of randomized controllled trials conducted with older adults. Maturitas-June2016.91:101-109 doi:http://dx.doi.org/10.1016/jmaturitas 2016.06.016

48. McGlade C, Daly E, Cornally N, Weathers E, O'Caoimh R, McCarthy J, Cronin U, Molloy D.W, Challenges in Implementing Advance Care Planning in Long Term Care Journal of Nursing Ethics (In press).

50. Kearns T, Cornally N, Molloy W. Patient Reported Outcome Measures of Quality of End-of-Life Care: A Systematic Review. Maturitas, 2016. DOI: http://dx.doi.org/10.1016/j.maturitas.2016.11.004.

ACKNOWLEDGEMENTS

Thanks to colleague and friend Mareeta Calnan for all her invaluable help and patience putting this together.

Special thanks to:
Ronan O'Sullivan, Dr. Roger Clarette, Dr Ronán ó Caoimh, Dr Ciara McGlade, Dr Kieran O'Connor, Dr Catherine O'Sullivan, Dr Nicola Cornally, Dr Carol Fitzgerald, Dr Edel Daly, Yvonne McCarthy, Dr Feargal Twomey, Ber Power, Neil McKay, Bruce Pierce, Minister Kathleen Lynch, Dr Ruth Halley, Dr Tara Kerins, Mary, June, Dick, Tom, John, Jim, and Alex.

Health Research Board, and University College Cork.

We are immensely grateful for the support of Atlantic Philanthropies in the realisation of this project.

All the staff at Haven Bay, Kinsale, St Colombanus, Killarney, and St Lukes, Cork.